T0195153

Psychotic Disorders

Psychotic Disorders

Comorbidity Detection Promotes Improved Diagnosis and Treatment

ANDRÉ BARCIELA VERAS, MD, PhD

Professor of Psychiatry
Department of Psychiatry
State University of Mato Grosso do Sul (UEMS)
Campo Grande, Mato Grosso do Sul, Brazil

JEFFREY PAUL KAHN, MD

Clinical Professor of Psychiatry
Department of Psychiatry
Weill-Cornell Medical College, Cornell University
New York, New York, USA

ELSEVIER

Elsevier
1600 John F. Kennedy Blvd.
Ste 1800
Philadelphia, PA 19103-2899

PSYCHOTIC DISORDERS: COMORBIDITY DETECTION
PROMOTES IMPROVED DIAGNOSIS AND TREATMENT   ISBN: 978-0-323-68309-8

Notice

International Standard Book Number: 978-0-323-68309-8

Content Strategist: Joslyn Chaiprasert-Paguio
Content Development Specialist: Kevin Travers
Publishing Services Manager: Deepthi Unni
Project Manager: Srividhya Vidhyashankar
Design Direction: Ryan Cook

Printed in United States of America

Last digit is the print number: 9   8   7   6   5   4   3   2   1

Working together
to grow libraries in
developing countries

www.elsevier.com • www.bookaid.org

Gilberto Sousa Alves Sr., MD, PhD
Translational Psychiatry Research Group,
Department of Medicine I, Federal University
of Maranhão, São Luís, Maranhão, Brazil
Post Graduate Program in Psychiatry and
Mental Health, Institute of Psychiatry, Federal
University of Rio de Janeiro, Rio de Janeiro,
Rio de Janeiro, Brazil

Aline França da Hora Amarães
Dom Bosco Catholic University
Campo Grande, Mato Grosso, do Sul, Brazil

Emeka Boka, MD, MBA
Clinical Research Coordinator, Psychiatry, Icahn
School of Medicine at Mount Sinai, New York,
New York, USA

Lucas Briand
Department of Internal Medicine
Federal University of Ceará
Fortaleza, Ceará, Brazil

Carolina Gomes Carrilho
Dom Bosco Catholic University, Campo
Grande, Mato Grosso, do Sul, Brazil

Sulaima Daboul, MD, MHA
Clinical Research Scholar, Psychiatry, Icahn
School of Medicine at Mount Sinai,
New York, New York, USA

Maria Rita Silva de Souza, BSc
Dom Bosco Catholic University,
Campo Grande, Mato Grosso, do Sul, Brazil

Rafael C. Freire, MD, PhD
Associate Professor, Department of Psychiatry,
Queen's University, Kingston, Ontario,
Canada
Adjunct Professor, Laboratory of Panic and
Respiration, Federal University of Rio de
Janeiro, Rio de Janeiro, Rio de Janeiro, Brazil

Tony P. George, MD
Professor of Psychiatry, Department of
Psychiatry, University of Toronto, Toronto,
Ontario, Canada

Michael Hwang, MD
Medical Director and Chairman
Department of Psychiatry
Health Alliance Hospital Kingston, New York
Professor of Clinical Psychiatry
New York Medical College
Valhalla, New York
New York, USA

Jeffrey Paul Kahn, MD
Clinical Professor of Psychiatry
Department of Psychiatry
Weill-Cornell Medical College, Cornell
University
New York, New York, USA

Fabiana Leão Lopes, MD, PhD
Human Genetics Branch
National Institute of Mental Health (NIHM)
Intramural Research Program
National Institutes of Health (NIH)
US Department of Health and Human Services
Bethesda, Maryland, USA

Darby J.E. Lowe, BSc
Addictions Division
CAMH and Institute of Medical Sciences
University of Toronto Toronto,
Ontario, Canada

Dolores Malaspina, MD, MS, MPH
Professor, Psychiatry Neuroscience &
Genetics, Psychiatry, Icahn School of
Medicine at Mount Sinai, New York, New
York, USA

Mariana Bonotto Mallmann, MSc, PhD
Dom Bosco Catholic University, Campo
Grande, Mato Grosso, do Sul, Brazil

Kethlyn Carolina, BSc
Dom Bosco Catholic University, Campo
Grande, Mato Grosso, do Sul, Brazil

Antonio E. Nardi, MD, PhD
Full Professor, Institute of Psychiatry, Federal
University of Rio de Janeiro, Rio de Janeiro,
Rio de Janeiro, Brazil

Michael Poyurovsky, MD
Tirat Carmel Mental Health Center
Department of First Episode Psychosis
Tirat Carmel, Israel

Laiana A. Quagliato, MD, MSc
Federal University of Rio de Janeiro,
Laboratory of Panic & Respiration, Institute
of Psychiatry, Rio de Janeiro, Brazil

Nadia Rahman
Clinical Research Coordinator
Psychiatry Icahn School of Medicine at
Mount Sinai New York
New York, USA

Thaysse Gomes Ricci, PhD
Dom Bosco Catholic University, Campo
Grande, Mato Grosso, do Sul, Brazil

Sarah-Maude Rioux
Addictions Division
CAMH
Department of Psychiatry
University of Toronto
Toronto, Ontario, Canada

Julia Sasiadek, BA
Addictions Division
CAMH and Institute of Medical Sciences
University of Toronto
Toronto, Ontario, Canada

Leandro Oliveira Trovão, MSc, MD, PhD
Translational Psychiatry Research Group
Federal University of Maranhão, Brazil

André Barciela Veras, MD, PhD
Professor of Psychiatry
Department of Psychiatry
State University of Mato Grosso do Sul (UEMS)
Campo Grande, Mato Grosso do Sul, Brazil

In recent years, there have been several specialist books on schizophrenia. This specialization is important since schizophrenia is so complex and reflects that our field is moving forward appropriately. All that said, such specialization also makes it hard for us as clinicians to maintain current in basic knowledge and treatment developments across so many facets of this enigmatic condition. Additionally, there has been a growing appreciation of the common occurrence of psychiatric and medical comorbidities in schizophrenia. There is a pressing need to evaluate and incorporate these comorbidities in determining treatment and broader functional outcomes in people with schizophrenia.

Accordingly, I am delighted that Drs Veras and Kahn have collaborated in assembling a group of leading international experts to author this book that will serve as an authoritative source on psychiatric comorbidities in schizophrenia. The style of the book, including brief "case reports" to exemplify key aspects of psychiatric comorbidities, will be particularly beneficial for mental health clinicians. The book covers the clinical essentials of each comorbidity - panic and social anxiety disorders, depressions, bipolar disorder, substance abuse, medical comorbidities in schizophrenia - in a balanced and comprehensive manner. Each chapter deals with a specific comorbidity in the contemporary manner that also incorporates the most current issues in schizophrenia research. Drs Veras and Kahn and their impressive cadre of contributing authors are also to be congratulated for including the very latest key publications while also citing references to seminal papers on each comorbidity in schizophrenia.

Finally, as the authors remind us throughout the book, each comorbidity holds substantial potential to advance our psychopathological understanding, treatments, and outcomes for patients with schizophrenia.

Peter F. Buckley, M
Interim Senior Vice President for VIrginia Commonwealth University (VCU)
Health Sciences and Interim Chief Executive Officer of VCU Health System
Dean, VCU School of Medicine Executive Vice President for Medical Affairs,
VCU Health System
Richmond
Virginia
USA

Psychiatrists have long wondered how best to divide psychotic disorders into meaningful and treatable subtypes. Past subtyping of schizophrenia has been of little clinical utility, and is now largely abandoned. This book proposes that there are five types of "functional" psychosis, each associated with a particular anxiety or depressive comorbidity, and three already well recognized (delusional disorder, delusional depression, bipolar I mania). In addition, psychoses can be caused or exacerbated by substance abuse and by medical illness and treatment. Co-morbidity diagnosis in psychosis is not an inconsequential effort. Although it can take time and effort, it results in improved treatment that has been shown to improve clinical outcome. In addition, the co-morbidities may be more than incidental syndromes. They typically precede psychosis onset, and may be part of the underlying psychosis process.

Much of recent research on psychotic disorders has focused on symptoms, genetics, imaging, and other methods to divine a newer subtyping approach. Many of these studies are cited here, including some that suggest a five-co-morbidity subtype model, with each co-morbidity superimposed upon a more global psychosis susceptibility factor. Indeed, the current DSM5 advises that all comorbidities be diagnosed and considered for treatment. Although these diagnoses can be difficult to ascertain in psychotic patients, focused diagnostic methods are included herein. The diagnosis and treatment model in this book derives largely from clinical practice and research, and from evolutionary theory, and also posits a central global psychosis proneness factor.

The theory began to take shape in chapter seven (psychosis) of Angst: Origins of Anxiety and Depression (Kahn JP, Oxford University Press, 2013). That book examined five core anxiety and depressive subtypes from evolutionary, clinical, research and ethological perspectives. The core theory was that anxiety and depression originated as altruistic primeval social instincts for evolutionary survival of the group, and despite distressing and dysfunctional effects on many individual members.

In modern humans, those primeval instincts are countered by conscious choices and by cultural influences, while our modern concepts of altruism may be quite different. Melancholic depression, Atypical Depression, Social anxiety, Panic anxiety and Obsessive-compulsive Disorder can be exacerbated by our modern personal agency, even as we succeed at goals that our primeval instincts painfully complain. An extensive research literature supported the general and the diagnosis-specific theories. Psychosis is seen in the earlier volume and in this one as the psychotic presentation of these five disorders. Psychosis emerges when psychosis proneness allows inborn primeval instinctive fears and behaviors to overwhelm our consciousness.

This approach may provide a foundation for better understanding the mechanisms, origins, subtyping, and treatment of the psychoses. Indeed, clinical experience and varying amounts of research appear to support the idea that appropriate medication for certain co-morbidities, along with anti-psychotic medication and skilled psychotherapy may effect substantially improved outcomes.

Your two editors are psychiatrists with decades of clinical practice and research. Research training in anxiety, combined with research and practice in psychotic disorders lead to their interest in co-morbidity interactions. One of us first published on alprazolam treatment of schizophrenia with panic anxiety in 1988. The other editor completed a PhD on the relationship of social anxiety and psychosis.

It is our fervent hope that this book will help mental health professionals to better understand the importance, diagnosis and treatment of psychosis co-morbidities. In addition to the substantial benefits for our patients, this approach may lead to further and more sophisticated research, deeper psychopathological understanding, and greater acceptance of this clinical perspective.

Andre Barciela Veras, MD, PhD
Adjunct Professor of Psychiatry
Medical School at the State University of Mato Grosso do Sul

Jeffrey Paul Kahn, MD
Clinical Professor of Psychiatry
Weill-Cornell Medical College, Cornell University

July 9, 2020

Disclaimer

The information in this book is not intended as a definitive assessment or treatment strategy, but as one suggested approach for clinicians treating patients with psychotic disorders. Diagnosis of the co-morbidity diagnoses is difficult during acute psychosis, somewhat easier after initiation of antipsychotic medication, and always essential. Co-morbidity diagnosis always requires a detailed, thorough and proactive assessment of internally experienced syndromes: outwardly obvious comorbidities are rarely apparent. Individual cases will vary and should be evaluated carefully before treatment is provided.

Medications noted are generally approved for the targeted co-morbidity. Though they are not generally approved for the psychosis itself, clinical and research experience suggest that they may benefit the psychosis as well. Some chapters discuss posited novel diagnostic categories based on a commonly associated co-morbidity. These have not all been proven or generally accepted. All cases in this book are fictional, though influenced by clinical experience.

Knowledge and best practice in this field are constantly changing. As new research and experience broaden our understanding, changes in research methods, professional practices, or medical treatment may become necessary. Practitioners and researchers must always rely on their own experience and knowledge in evaluating and using any information, methods, compounds or experiments described herein.

Because of rapid advances in the medical sciences, in particular, independent verification of diagnoses and drug dosages should be made. To the fullest extent of the law, no responsibility is assumed by Elsevier, authors, editors or contributors for any injury and/or damage to persons or property as a matter of products liability, negligence or otherwise, or from any use or operation of any methods, products, instructions, or ideas contained in the material herein.

ACKNOWLEDGMENTS

We are delighted to offer the results of our Pan-American endeavor to the psychiatric and mental health communities. With editors based in Rio de Janeiro and New York, this volume drew inspiration from research and researchers around the world.

Our South American institutions included the Psychiatric Institute of the Federal University of Rio de Janeiro, originally named the Psychiatric Institute of the University of Brazil (IPUB-UFRJ). The first Brazilian psychiatric hospital was built there in 1842. Here, too, arose the seminal psychopathological contributions of José Leme Lopes (1904-1990), as well as the research activities of the current chair professor of psychiatry, Dr. Antonio Egidio Nardi. Both editors offer a special thank you to Dr. Nardi for his mentorship, guidance, support, friendship, and enablement of our collaborations past and present. From Rio, other professors that strongly influenced the psychiatric perspective of this book include Marcia Rozenthal, Márcio Versiani, Maria Tavares, and Alexandre Valença. Besides the Federal University of Rio de Janeiro, research grant support was provided by the Brazilian federal agencies CAPES and CNPq, and institutional support by the Dom Bosco Catholic University, and by the Medical School at the State University of Mato Grosso do Sul, the present academic home of our South American editor. Carolina Gomes Carrilho, was a brilliant collaborator a co-manager, resolving so many important and time-sensitive tasks.

Inspirations from North America are wide ranging within the United States and Canada. Our New York editor developed his psychiatric thinking at Columbia under the teaching and guidance of Roger MacKinnon (interview skills, phenomenology), Donald Klein (psychopathology, psychopharmacology, research methodology, attention to unfamiliar details), and Robert Spitzer (diagnostic criteria and DSM). Earlier skills were learned at Albert Einstein College of Medicine from researchers Wagner Bridger and Edward Sachar. But most importantly, the co-morbidity approach of this book was helped by faculty colleagues, students and patients at Weill-Cornell Medical College, his current academic home. Psychiatry Chairman Francis Lee and Jack Barchas before him have been helpful and supportive. Clinical practice with thousands of patients, and clinical teaching with hundreds more allowed for careful contemplation of clinical phenomenology and treatment effectiveness. More than a hundred psychotic patients seen in clinical teaching allowed medical students to learn the complexities and importance of psychiatric diagnosis.

This project would never have moved forward without the encouragement and expert editorial guidance of Kevin Travers and Joslyn Chaiprasert-Paguio at Elsevier. Nor could it have been completed without the effort and expertise of our chapter authors.

Finally, we are indebted to our two Pan-American families, whose patient support has been essential, and whose tolerance of the time requirements has been gracious. Our two Pan-American continents, medical schools and collaboration have led to wonderful meals, intellectual discourse, vigorous discussion of the merits of Brazilian cachaça and Kentucky bourbon, and a close bond of friendship.

CONTENTS

CHAPTER 1

Introduction: Diagnosing Comorbidity Trees in the Forest of Psychosis

Carolina Gomes Carrilho   ▓   André Barciela Veras   ▓   Jeffrey Paul Kahn

Abstract

Despite so many false starts over the years, there are currently several well-recognized and distinct subtypes of psychosis. These subtypes allow differential determination of clinical course, prognosis, and especially of optimal treatment. Part of what allowed this progress was attention to the psychiatric and medical comorbidities of psychosis. From delusional depression to medical illness, there is strong evidence for the value of treating those comorbidities as well. This volume offers an overview of psychoses and their comorbidities and also looks at more recently accumulating research, clinical experience, and conceptual frameworks. Although not all comorbidities serve to define a psychosis subtype, some of those more recently studied may be associated with proposed additions to psychotic diagnoses. All comorbidities have significant potential value for improving treatment, outcome, and psychopathologic understanding. Converging concepts from data analytic studies and from evolutionary theory suggest that there may be five core functional psychoses, as well as others due to substance use and to medical illness and treatment.

KEYWORDS

Psychosis	Comorbidities	Differential diagnosis
Transdiagnostic	Evolutionary theory	Ultra-high risk
Psychopathology		

Definition of Functional Psychosis

Primeval social instincts helped safeguard both ancient human groups and modern animal groups of all kinds, but we humans also have an evolutionary advantage when it comes to consciousness. That ability to think about thinking has helped us evaluate environmental and interpersonal situations, readapt, reorganize environments, and inform our social interactions and other needs. So, conscious reason has allowed humans to adapt and prosper beyond the reach of other species. Our consciousness instinct is responsible for moderating our primeval social instincts.[1] However, a decrease of that rational consciousness can allow the reemergence of instinctual perceptions and beliefs, leading to heightened prominence of social instincts and to frightening concerns.

With consciousness, we humans can overcome biological social instincts, and we can better rely on reasoning to achieve better outcomes in both challenging and promising situations.

1

Consciousness and self-awareness are adaptive traits that can improve human life when focused on ourselves and especially when focused on others. However, when consciousness decreases and social instincts emerge, we have a loss of contact with reality and with normal social functioning. When extreme, these unmoderated socially instinctive beliefs can be called "psychosis," as in the overused but paradigmatically termed "schizophrenia."

Eugene Bleuler (1857–1939) described "The Group of Schizophrenias" with a presumed biological cause. Considering how our inner unconscious holds much of our social instinct, it is remarkable that Bleuler, in coining the term "schizophrenia" in 1908, understood it as an illness where the brain splits apart between a conscious mind (think conscious reason) and an inner unconscious (think social instinct), so that the inner unconscious then dominates. Although primeval social instincts are adaptive to a point even today, when they are too dominant, they can contribute to psychotic experiences.[1]

Psychosis is a clinical category with various symptoms, and diagnosis is possible only through psychotic clinical manifestations, rather than through laboratory, genetic, and neuroimaging investigation.[2] According to the American Psychiatric Association's (2013) Diagnostic and Statistical Manual of Mental Disorders (5th ed.; DSM-5), psychotic features are defined by such alterations as delusions, hallucinations, disorganized thinking or speech, disorganized or abnormal motor behavior, and negative symptoms.[3]

Although psychosis includes a spectrum of several disorders, schizophrenia is only approximately 30% of the psychotic spectrum. Even so, it has been 10 times more researched than the other 70% of psychotic disorders. In clinical practice and public awareness, the term "schizophrenia" has been used to epitomize the nature of all psychosis types, even those with brief psychotic episodes, and those considered at ultra-high risk (UHR) for schizophrenia. And because schizophrenia is a chronic and progressive disorder, many professionals prefer to substitute diagnoses that suggest a better clinical outcome. Indeed, when psychotic patients do recover substantially, they are usually considered ineligible for the chronic diagnosis called schizophrenia.[4]

In the early editions of the Diagnostic and Statistical Manual of Mental Disorders, psychosis was defined more by the presence of functional limitations than by the role of symptoms in those limitations. Nowadays, schizophrenia diagnosis is made solely based on the presence of hallucinations and/or delusions without insight (i.e., by impairment of reality testing). However, there are other psychotic symptoms also commonly found in nonpsychotic patients that seem to affect severity, intensity, and the co-occurrence of hallucinations and delusions. These can include disorganized thinking, neologism, thought blocking, other disturbances of thought, and negative symptoms. It is also common for adolescents with psychosis to present anxiety, mood changes, and social withdrawal before the onset of the first psychotic episode, which can further explain the relation between nonpsychotic affective symptoms with thought disturbances and the more severe psychotic symptoms.[5,6]

Alongside psychotic symptoms, patients frequently have other psychiatric comorbidities. Missed diagnoses, and misdiagnoses are also common, despite the seeming homogeneity of psychotic disorders.[6] The core diagnoses in nonpsychotic patients are also the most common comorbidities in schizophrenia: melancholic major depression, atypical major depression, obsessive-compulsive disorder, panic disorder, and social anxiety. In addition, these comorbidities can worsen prognosis and increase symptom severity; therefore adequate diagnosis and treatment of comorbidities can ameliorate positive and negative psychotic symptoms.[7]

A History of Psychosis Differential Diagnosis

Psychosis derives from the Greek word "*psykhe*" (mind) and "*osis*" (diseased state), which means mental disorder. The term "psychosis" was used to explain interactions between physical and mental processes. A German pathologist and neurologist named Nikolaus Friedreich (1825–1882) thought of psychosis as a combination of physical brain anomality and mental vulnerability, with a predominantly organic neurologic basis. Therefore psychosis was used to explain "insanity" and "mental illness."[8]

Emil Kraepelin (1856–1926) explained how different diseases had similar processes and would produce similar symptoms, pathologic anatomy, and common etiology. People believed each disorder had its own etiology, pathologic anatomy, and symptoms, but Kraepelin believed many disorders had similar symptoms and biological foundations that would follow different courses as illness progressed. He then grouped illnesses such as catatonia, hebephrenia, and dementia paranoides into one condition called "dementia praecox," with the idea that this illness was present in young people and had symptoms such as inappropriate emotions, stereotyped behavior, distraction or confusion, hallucinations, irrational beliefs or delusions, and a deterioration of mental functions.[8]

Besides dementia praecox, Kraepelin also differentiated dementia praecox from manic depressive illnesses and paranoia, the last two with better prognoses. Manic depressive illnesses were mood disorders, whereas paranoia had symptoms of delusional belief with less severity than in dementia praecox. Inspired in part by Kraepelin's work, Bleuler then coined the term "schizophrenia," believing dementia praecox did not adequately define psychosis. His notion of schizophrenia was a pathologic splitting apart of the emotional and rational consciousness parts of psychic functioning. Catatonia, which was once apart from dementia praecox classification by Kraepelin, was then included within schizophrenia.[8] A psychiatrist named Jacob Kasanin (1897–1946) coined the term "schizoaffective disorder," to reflect symptoms of schizophrenia, mood disorders such as mania and depression, and hallucinations, but with fewer symptoms of passivity.[8]

Just as depressive symptoms can vary in number and severity, there are patients with only a few psychosis-related symptoms but not enough to diagnose a psychotic disorder. A psychosis continuum supposition would encompass the range of psychosis symptom variety and severity in the general population. This range includes the overt psychoses, as well as many people with minor symptoms that can include hallucinations, delusions, and ideas of reference. For example, benign hypnogogic hallucinations typically include a voice calling someone's name as they fall off to sleep. Because psychosis has several symptom dimensions that overlap with affective and nonaffective disorders, it could be thought of as both an illness continuum and also a heterogeneous disorder.[9]

DSM's diagnostic criteria for schizophrenia are clinically relevant and useful; however, it does not provide essential information about the nature, etiology, biology, social aspects, risk factors, and structure of schizophrenia. Many professionals have debated the construct validity of schizophrenia, in view of psychotic-like experiences in many other psychotic and nonpsychotic disorders, and even in the normal population.[10]

Current Psychosis Differential Diagnostic Theories

Dopamine-blocking antipsychotic medication treatment has been used for nearly 70 years. Medications that block the effect of dopamine can decrease positive symptoms in all psychotic patients, leading to the realization that all forms of psychosis are somehow related to an increase in dopamine activity. This observation led to the dopamine theory of schizophrenia, and later genetic and epigenetic research further increased our understanding.[1] Although antipsychotics have not shown greatly improved efficacy over time, successive medication generations have had milder side effect profiles than previous antipsychotics. However, studies have not shown whether the increase of dopamine in psychosis is related to an excess of dopamine, an excess of dopamine receptors, a hypersensitivity to dopamine, or a combination of those and other factors.[11]

Individuals with subclinical psychotic features tend to show increased dopamine synthesis capacity. But this increased capacity is only among those who later develop overt psychosis.

Increased dopamine synthesis capacity is also associated with severity in psychotic disorders. An increase in dopamine levels is also more commonly found in people who are acutely psychotic, by comparison to people with more stable psychosis. Although higher serum dopamine levels are related to severity in schizophrenia, they are not specific to this disorder, and are present in the whole psychosis spectrum, including subclinical psychotic symptoms.[5]

Dopamine, as part of our reward and limbic systems, increases our satisfaction of appetitive instincts and makes us search for more satisfaction, pleasure, and inspiration. However, it is also responsible for increasing our ability to remember aversive situations, helping us recognize potentially dangerous situations and people, and thus amplifies our fear response. Because intense dopamine activation can intensely stimulate our primeval social instincts, that may diminish the role of our rational conscious thoughts. Faced with great pleasure just out of reach, many people will take reckless steps despite their better judgment. In sum, dopamine is responsible for increasing pleasure and appetites, as well as our fear or anger, supplementing the influence of our conscious rational thoughts.[1]

Dopamine abnormalities are common in both people with schizophrenia and people at high risk of psychosis, and the blocking of dopamine can reduce severity of prodromal symptoms in individuals at high risk. Dopamine synthesis capacity is also increased in individuals at clinical high risk for psychosis, which can cause greater severity of prodromal symptoms. Therefore neuroimaging studies have shown a link between dopaminergic dysfunction in schizophrenia prodrome with the clinical development of the disorder, thus suggesting a possible causal role.[12]

Consciousness is thought to occur in the frontal cortex. The hypofrontality theory of schizophrenia points to a thinning of the frontal cortex that is found both in people with psychosis and in people at high risk for schizophrenia. Because frontal lobe thinning is present before schizophrenia onset and is not later linked to severity or duration of illness, it is not a consequence or result of the illness. Diminished frontal lobe function impairs conscious thought, reduces attention span, and impedes processing of social cues. Similar to Bleuler's notion of schizophrenia, psychosis may result from this imbalance of consciousness and socially instinctive emotions.[1]

Neuroimaging studies have shown great progress in understanding the neurologic aspects of psychosis. In laboratory neuroimaging studies, people with schizophrenia have shown decreased brain activity and changes in the neuroanatomy of the cerebral hemisphere. This can help explain their decreased ability to understand the intent underlying a human action, to recognize pictures they have already seen, and to explain difficulties with abstract thought. These decreased abilities and cognitive impairments are also present in patients with mood-related disorders and individuals at high risk of schizophrenia.[1,13]

Since frontal lobe executive function is correlated with both clinical insight and cognitive insight, the cognitive impairment of psychosis results in impaired insight.[14,15] In general, people at high risk for schizophrenia have poor conscious processing of social and emotional information, facial expressions, and social interactions. This is also shown by their need for intensified brain activity when given theory-of-mind tests (the ability to assess others' thoughts and emotional state) and further points to diminished consciousness well before the onset of psychosis.[1]

Nonpsychotic people with increased dopaminergic activity or with cerebral cortex hypofrontality are more prone to develop psychosis and are more likely to transition from nonpsychotic anxiety or depressive disorder to a psychotic form. Comorbid anxiety or depressive syndromes may be directly related to diagnostic subtyping of psychosis. Ordinary anxiety disorders that evoke weak quasipsychotic symptoms suggest some overlap between nonpsychotic and psychotic categories and support the psychosis spectrum approach. From this point of view, developmental factors can help determine the severity level along the spectrum. Not surprisingly, minor psychotic symptoms in early life can help predict later psychosis, and untreated comorbidities can increase this risk.[7,16]

A neurodevelopmental hypothesis of psychosis posits that prenatal and perinatal events can increase the risk for psychosis by interaction with structural brain defects.[5] Indeed, some genetic features of schizophrenia are shown during fetal development, predicting compromised cognitive development in early adult life and later psychotic illness.[17] At the same time, neurodevelopmental hypotheses suggest that the low cognitive performance of people with schizophrenia may also correlate with other prenatal and perinatal risk factors or genetic factors. The cognitive impairment in schizophrenia is determined by a complex interaction of nature, nurture, and the illness itself.[18]

Illustrating this complex interaction, patients with schizophrenia who have more early risk factors show greater sensitivity to everyday trauma in comparison with controls, which in turn can then worsen psychotic symptoms and increase psychosis severity. A comprehensive neurodevelopmental theory would explain not only how biological risk and genetic factors can make someone's brain more prone to psychosis but also how that risk interacts with psychological development, social environment, and both emotionally and physiologically significant events. The overall sum of these effects determines psychotic disorder occurrence and severity, as well as comorbidities.[16]

Murray et al.[16] highlights a vicious cycle in psychosis where stress can increase dopamine dysregulation, which causes psychotic experiences with yet more stress, and finally more dopamine release. This hypothesis has created a new model emerging from the neurodevelopmental model: The developmental risk factor model, which sees schizophrenia as the severe end of a broad multidimensional psychosis spectrum. Thus the psychosis spectrum would encompass a continuum of subclinical psychotic symptoms that can be present in the general population in different levels of severity and reoccurrence.

Evolutionary Theory and the Group of Schizophrenias

Evolution selects for adaptive genes. Those adaptive genes are contained in DNA and act to increase the likelihood of its own replication and survival in the population gene pool. However, given that psychotic disorders generally lead to fewer descendants, why haven't psychosis-prone genes disappeared over time? One theory is that, although overt psychosis leads to fewer children, milder versions have some sort of kin group survival and reproductive value. Looking at this from a psychosis spectrum point of view: persecutory delusional disorder (associated with social anxiety) may reduce reproduction, but social anxiety can include mildly psychosis-like oversensitivity to potentially dangerous people.[19] In addition, there may be other kin group adaptive benefits to a mild reduction in rational consciousness. Randolph Nesse[20] refers to the transition point of overt psychosis as the "cliff-edge" of reproductive failure.

The evolved social instincts mentioned earlier primarily have a primeval altruistic value for humans and other species. They are instinctive prompts for social behaviors that may be evolutionarily adaptive for the kin group but often conflict with the perceptions and social values of rational consciousness and modern civilization. The genes behind those instincts have survived because they are adaptive for the kin group as a whole. They still underly our overall perception and behavior, and for affected individuals, they sometimes tend to cause emotional pain and reproductive disadvantage. Primeval instinctive altruism differs greatly from modern conscious altruism.

When psychosis proneness diminishes consciousness, primeval instincts can emerge in their unmodified primeval form. Along the lines of Bleuler's "group of schizophrenias," each of the five primeval social instincts may determine a specific psychotic disorder comorbidity, or even specific psychosis subtypes. Diagnosis and treatment of the comorbidities can greatly improve clinical outcome. Those five psychosis-associated disorders are the core of this book, briefly reviewed below in this introduction.

Recent research has taken a "transdiagnostic" look at psychotic disorders. Largely through statistical analysis of psychosis rating scales, at least two studies suggest that there are five psychosis subtypes, as well as a separate factor for psychosis proneness. This resembles the clinically transdiagnostic approach of this volume, with five subtypes and psychosis proneness as the key determinants of more specific and more treatable psychosis subtypes.[21,22] Although direct comparison of those two sets of five statistical subtypes to the five clinical subtypes in this volume is not yet possible, there is at least face plausibility that they could coincide with the five subtypes here.[1,7]

Evolutionary theory must ultimately agree with genetic research findings. Thus genetics has found hundreds of gene variants associated with schizophrenia but has had limited success in finding genes for endophenotypes. There has been greater success in finding genes associated with psychosis proneness. One possibility is that genes interact with developmental, environmental, and other factors either epigenetically or otherwise. These secondary forces make finding underlying genes more elusive or less specific.[23] Then again, the endophenotypes may be genetically influenced by genes for the five associated comorbidities.

Transdiagnostic study of symptoms could mean that working on a single symptom can also ameliorate related downstream symptoms, if they are linked through a causal chain.[23] Moreover, understanding psychosis through a transdiagnostic dimension can allow greater comprehension of multifaceted symptoms and their underlying dynamics. Although psychosis is sometimes considered mostly schizophrenia, current researchers again think that there are a variety of psychotic experiences.[24]

Psychosis may be related to other psychiatric disorders and is not exclusively schizophrenia, and milder symptoms can appear in nonpsychotic disorders. When exacting diagnosis and newer subtypes are taken into account, it is even possible that schizophrenia will be mostly redefined as a collection of well-defined psychotic subtypes.[24,25]

Establishing clear definitions and criteria for those subtypes has many potential benefits. Diagnostically, it would improve diagnostic criteria and precision, as well as knowledge of clinical phenomenology. For research, it would enhance genetic, epidemiologic, neuroimaging, psychotherapeutic, and psychopharmacologic approaches. Most importantly, clinical treatment of subtypes and associated comorbidities will allow greatly improved treatment and outcome. The transdiagnostic approach can have a huge impact on how we view and deal with mental illness, once related comorbidities, such as mood and anxiety disorders, are seen as core syndromes rather than as a hodgepodge of secondary distress symptoms.[23,26,27] Many studies have shown a high prevalence of mood and anxiety disorders associated with psychosis spectrum disorders.

Obsessive-compulsive disorder (OCD; Chapter 3) is one common comorbidity. Obsessive and compulsive symptoms are often present prior to psychosis onset, often starting in childhood. Similarly, OCD symptoms associate with earlier age of psychosis onset, as well as diminished functioning in psychotic patients.[7] Comorbid obsessive-compulsive symptoms correlate with increased schizophrenia severity, obsessions, mind-reading concerns, and inappropriate sexual impulses. As noted in the OCD chapter, criteria for a "schizo-obsessive disorder" have been proposed.

Panic disorder (Chapter 4) is also a common comorbidity in schizophrenia, occurring in 7.1% to 47.5% of schizophrenia patients, and panic attacks are often masked when they are component parts of psychotic symptoms. Sometimes, panic anxiety precedes and triggers such psychotic symptoms as auditory hallucinations and paranoid delusions. When psychosis-masked panic is closely evaluated, the panic comorbidity in schizophrenia with voices may be 100%.[28] In addition, panic is also associated with guilty delusions, which can be found in nonpsychotic anxiety disorders as well. As noted in the Panic chapter, although a panic psychosis has been proposed, much research remains to be done.[1]

Social anxiety (Chapter 5) is also associated with schizophrenia generally and with delusional disorder in particular. Social anxiety correlates with paranoia, social withdrawal, feelings of inadequacy, negative assessment by others, and mind reading in both patients with schizophrenia and with persecutory delusional disorder. This can also cause symptoms of mind reading and socialphobic delusions of negative assessment.[7]

Depression in psychosis is commonly associated with greater positive and negative symptoms. Depressive symptoms are also common with earlier psychosis onset, and both can diminish coping and heighten psychotic experience.

Melancholic depression (Chapter 6) another specific depressive subtype, may underly psychotic (delusional) depression. This syndrome includes greater psychological distress, feelings of guilt and victimization, and persecutory delusions. As noted in its chapter, this subtype has long been formally established, and dual treatment of depression and psychosis are typically the best treatment.[7]

Atypical depression (Chapter 7) a specific depressive subtype, is the most common depression in true bipolar I disorder. Mania, with its delusions of grandeur, can be considered a psychosis, and it is often misdiagnosed as schizophrenia. Mania is associated with certain markers of psychosis-proneness. In addition, some manic patients have auditory hallucinations and more elaborated delusions. However, mania is a recurrent component, whereas atypical depression is an ongoing illness. The association of the two has no well-defined mechanism. Even so, manic delusions are typically focused on saving the world, while the rejection sensitivity of atypical depression leads to avoidance of offensive behavior, thus saving social harmony.

With these five subtypes in mind, as well as those psychoses related to substance abuse (Chapter 8) and to medical illness and treatment (Chapter 9), the evolutionary and transdiagnostic perspective can allow us to better understand and individually treat each patient. Psychosis is not a specific and unitary disorder with variable symptoms. Rather, there are several overlapping symptoms related to nonpsychotic disorders. This perspective can help professionals avoid treat overt psychotic symptoms, while also addressing those contributory comorbid syndromes that can aggravate or cause psychosis.[1,7]

Psychosis and Mixed Comorbidities

Isolated psychotic experiences found in nonpsychotic patients have been typically found in patients with anxiety or depression and may even occur in the general population, ranging in prevalence from 0.6% to 84%.[29,30] These experiences are often related to psychiatric disorder severity and poor treatment outcome. Therefore, if psychotic experiences can worsen prognosis, it is beneficial to understand how symptoms interact, to clarify diagnostic criteria.[24]

Although disorders are organized through symptoms and clusters, each patient will manifest them in different ways. This broad range of symptom manifestations, the ability to find those symptoms in the general population, and the overlap of symptoms in different disorders can hinder and cloud diagnosis. So, it is extremely common for people within the psychosis spectrum to have affective symptoms, as it is common for people with mood disorders to have different but overlapping affective symptoms and present such manifestations of other disorders as psychotic symptoms and anxiety.[23]

Patients with schizophrenia often present comorbidities such as obsessive-compulsive disorder, social anxiety, depression, and other anxiety disorders. Many of these disorders occur at a rate higher in schizophrenia than in the general population. And, just as nonpsychotic patients with one of these syndromes often have more than one, the same phenomenon of multiple comorbidities occurs in schizophrenia. That makes full and accurate diagnosis more important and more confusingly difficult.

It is common for schizophrenia patients to have panic anxiety, which tends to begin before schizophrenia onset.[7] Higher panic anxiety levels make patients more likely to hear more voices and have more delusions, just as nonpsychotic patients with panic disorder have increased brain activity to experimental noise. Emerging data suggest that voices usually occur together with panic symptoms in patients with psychosis.[1,27]

Although not categorized as a symptom for a psychosis diagnosis, cognitive biases such as jumping to conclusions (JTC) and liberal acceptance (seeking less information to reach a decision) are associated with psychosis and delusions; they are also seen in other psychiatric disorders with delusion-like experiences. This implies a transdiagnostic process, where cognitive biases may have a role in forming delusions.[23,31]

In addition, individuals at UHR for schizophrenia show higher than normal rates of depression and anxiety, and conversely, psychotic-like experiences are more common in individuals with anxiety and depressive disorders.[26] Some research points to melancholic and atypical major depression, obsessive-compulsive disorder, panic disorder, and social anxiety as the five core diagnoses in nonpsychotic patients and commonly found in schizophrenia as both single and multiple comorbidities.[7]

Depressive symptoms in schizophrenia may be associated with diminished coping, heightened psychotic experiences, greater psychological distress while deluded or hallucinating, and the obsessional guilt and victimization commonly found in delusional depression. These may also increase risk for suicide when compared with patients with nonpsychotic depression, and especially during the most acute phase of the illness.[7,32] Studies show that depression is often found in UHR individuals with nonpsychotic comorbid mental disorder at baseline.[33]

OCD can also increase schizophrenia severity with ego-dystonic obsessive delusions of aggressive, sexual, or guilt content and formal thought disorder of mind reading. Panic is also related to guilty delusions, as well as increased suicidal ideation, auditory hallucinations, early onset, and hospitalization. Lastly, social anxiety can be associated with social-phobic delusions of negative assessments and decrease in social anxiety instincts by the hypofrontality common in psychosis.[7]

A study investigating clinical outcomes of UHR patients ($N = 74$) at 6-year follow-up found that 28% of the UHR patients transitioned to psychosis and 56.8% presented at least one nonpsychotic comorbid mental disorder.[33] UHR patients with affective symptoms have better prognosis when treatments aim at reducing not only psychotic symptoms but also mood and anxiety symptoms. Therefore psychosis might arise from nonpsychotic subthreshold psychopathology that can develop into a more severe disorder under some circumstances.[34]

Although it is likely that comorbidity diagnostic assessment is often hindered by cognitive impairment, the effort is worthwhile. The ability to define psychosis comorbidities can help professionals differentiate among treatable and discrete syndromes. In turn, this helps to improve prognosis with more accurate and specific diagnoses that focus on psychosis, as well as on comorbidities. Recognition of the comorbidities requires awareness that they can both precede and coincide with psychotic processes.[7]

To work preventively in psychosis, professionals must be able to identify UHR patients and develop a holistic strategy to predict illness onset, early course, and subsequent evolution. The different comorbidities that can precede and coincide with psychosis may have different outcomes and pathways. UHR patients usually already have at least one comorbid diagnosis, such as anxiety or depressive disorders. In addition to other contributing factors, these early syndromes can also be part of a negative feedback loop. Anxiety and depression can decrease functional levels, causing more distress, thus aggravating themselves toward a psychotic outcome.[33,35]

Basic Interview Guidelines for Acutely Psychotic Patients

Diagnostic interviews of psychotic patients are not always easy and are more difficult still during acute psychosis. With that in mind, some basic guidelines can improve the odds of obtaining detailed and accurate symptom and syndrome history. Each of the diagnosis chapters in this book includes some additional guidelines specific to the different psychotic and comorbid diagnoses.

Because not every guideline is appropriate for every patient and interview, each suggestion should be considered in the context of each particular patient and interview. That said, here are some basic guidelines for interviewing actively psychotic patients:

- Be friendly, supportive, and professionally detached
- Too friendly or emotionally close can be threatening
- Emphasize and explain evaluation process and confidentiality rules
- Recruit a family member who may retain some of the patient's trust
- Everyone should avoid words such as "paranoid," "psychotic," "crazy," etc.
- Be honest, but carefully phrase questions and comments
- Start with a bit of small talk
- Then proceed to less emotionally loaded material (i.e., medical history, living arrangements, work history)
- Neither contradict nor agree with psychotic beliefs
- Recognize patient's point of view and perceived circumstances, even if psychotic
- Usually express empathic concern about their difficult situation
- Clinical knowledge of their diagnostic construct also shows empathy
- Some patients will slowly develop some fragile trust and open up a bit
- Always review both prepsychotic and psychotic history for comorbidities
- Review all symptoms of each psychotic and nonpsychotic syndrome considered
- Always carefully assess potential violence and self-harm risk
- In some cases, consider a weapons check
- Always remember that there may be unrevealed symptoms
- Conduct interview in a secure setting safe for patient and yourself
- Medication can be accurately proposed as an aid to their perceived struggle
- Usually repeat the diagnostic interview after acute psychosis is diminished

Summary: Limitations of Existing Research, Increasing Research Interest

Schizophrenia has long been seen as a collection of psychotic disorders. Various subtyping methods have been proposed and discarded over time. Meanwhile, at least three functional subtypes have been recognized as separate and distinct conditions: psychotic depression, delusional disorder, and bipolar I mania. Even so, those three conditions are often mislabeled as schizophrenia when the haze of patient psychosis and limited evaluation time combine to make specific subtyping difficult. Each of the three appears to have a commonly comorbid condition, while two more novel psychoses may also have comorbid determinants (obsessive-compulsive schizophrenia and panic psychosis). In addition, there are psychoses associated with substance abuse and with medical illness and treatment.

Alas, only some of this diagnostic schema are fully established, and much research remains, although it is clear that the comorbidities are common in psychoses. However, few genetic and neuroimaging studies used these comorbidities as markers to look for differing physiopathology in schizophrenia. Similarly, although psychotic-like experiences are included as markers for UHR for schizophrenia, studies do not usually evaluate anxiety and depressive subtypes, nor do they associate these syndromes with risk or phenomenology of schizophrenia. Longitudinal studies that follow up the symptom transformation from nonpsychotic to psychosis may be a frontier for new understanding of psychopathology and methods to avoid psychotic evolution. Finally, the study of comorbidities hidden among psychotic symptoms has been of increasing clinical interest. What is anecdotally clear to some clinicians is the vital importance of diagnosing and treating those comorbidities at the same time as the psychosis itself.

References

1. Kahn JP. *Angst: Origins of depression and anxiety*. New York: Oxford University Press; 2013.
2. Gaebel W, Zielasek J. Focus on psychosis. *Dialogues in Clinical Neuroscience*. 2015;17(1):9–18. 25987859.
3. American Psychiatric Association. *Diagnostic and statistical manual of mental disorders*. 5th ed. Arlington, VA: Author; 2013.
4. Guloksuz S, Van Os J. The slow death of the concept of schizophrenia and the painful birth of the psychosis spectrum. *Psychological Medicine*. 2018;48(2):229–244. https://doi.org/10.1017/S0033291717001775.
5. Howes OD, Murray RM. Schizophrenia: an integrated sociodevelopmental-cognitive model. *Lancet*. 2014;383(9929):1677–1687. https://doi.org/10.1016/S0140-6736(13)62036-X.
6. Arciniegas DB. Psychosis. *Continuum (Minneap Minn)*. 2015;21(3):715–736. https://doi.org/10.1212/01.CON.0000466662.89908.e7.
7. Veras AB, Cougo S, Meira F, Peixoto C, Barros JA, Nardi AE, et al. Schizophrenia dissection by five anxiety and depressive subtype comorbidities: clinical implications and evolutionary perspective. *Psychiatry Research*. 2017;257:172–178. https://doi.org/10.1016/j.psychres.2017.07.048.
8. Farrell M. *Psychosis under discussion: How we talk about madness*. London and New York: Routledge; 2018.
9. Murray RM, Jones PB, Sussere E, Van Os J, Cannon M. *The epidemiology of schizophrenia*. New York, NY: Cambridge University Press; 2003.
10. Tamminga CA, Sirovatka PJ, Regier DA, Van Os J. *Deconstructing psychosis: Refining the research agenda for DSM-V*. Arlington, VA: American Psychiatric Association; 2009.
11. Kaplan H, Sadock B, Grebb J. *Compêndio de Psiquiatria: Ciência do comportamento e psiquiatria clínica*. 9th ed. Porto Alegre: Artes Médicas; 2017.
12. Howes OD, McCutcheon R, Owen MJ, Murray RM. The role of genes, stress, and dopamine in the development of schizophrenia. *Biological Psychiatry*. 2017;81(1):9–20. https://doi.org/10.1016/j.biopsych.2016.07.014.
13. Mubarik A, Tohid H. Frontal lobe alterations in schizophrenia: a review. *Trends in Psychiatry and Psychotherapy*. 2016;38(4):198–206. https://doi.org/10.1590/2237-6089-2015-0088.
14. Bora E. Relationship between insight and theory of mind in schizophrenia: a meta-analysis. *Schizophrenia Research*. 2017;190:11–17. https://doi.org/10.1016/j.schres.2017.03.029.
15. Nair A, Palmer EC, Aleman A, David AS. Relationship between cognition, clinical and cognitive insight in psychotic disorders: a review and meta-analysis. *Schizophrenia Research*. 2014;152(1):191–200. https://doi.org/10.1016/j.schres.2013.11.033.
16. Murray RM, Bhavssar V, Tripoli G, Howes O. 30 Years on: How the neurodevelopmental hypothesis of schizophrenia morphed into the developmental risk factor model of psychosis. *Schizophrenia Bulletin*. 2017;43(6):1190–1196. https://doi.org/10.1093/schbul/sbx121.
17. Kahn RS, Sommer IE, Murray RM, Meyer-Lindenberg A, Weinberger DR, Cannon TD, et al. Schizophrenia Nature *Reviews Disease Primers*. 2015;1:15067. https://doi.org/10.1038/nrdp.2015.67.
18. Chua SE, Murray RM. The neurodevelopmental theory of schizophrenia: evidence concerning structure and neuropsychology. *Annals of Medicine*. 1996;28(6):547–555. https://doi.org/10.3109/07853899608999119.
19. Kim SY, Shin JE, Lee YI, Kim H, Jo HJ, Choi SH. Neural evidence for persistent attentional bias to threats in patients with social anxiety disorder. *Social Cognitive and Affective Neuroscience*. 2018;13(12):1327–1336.
20. Nesse RN. Cliff-edged fitness functions and the persistence of schizophrenia. *Behavioral and Brain Sciences*. 2004;27(6):862–863.
21. Anderson KK, Norman R, MacDougall A, Edwards J, Palaniyappan L, Lau C, Kurdyak P. Effectiveness of early psychosis intervention: comparison of service users and nonusers in population-based health administrative data. *The American Journal of Psychiatry*. 2018;175(5):443–452. https://doi.org/10.1176/appi.ajp.2017.17050480.
22. Quattrone D, Di Forti M, Gayer-Anderson C, Ferraro L, Jongsma HE, Tripoli G, et al. Transdiagnostic dimensions of psychopathology at first episode psychosis: findings from the multinational EU-GEI study. *Psychological Medicine*. 2019;49(8):1378–1391. https://doi.org/10.1017/S0033291718002131.
23. Bebbington P, Freeman D. Transdiagnostic extension of delusions: schizophrenia and beyond. *Schizophrenia Bulletin*. 2017;43(2):273–282. https://doi.org/10.1093/schbul/sbw191.
24. Van Os J. The transdiagnostic dimension of psychosis: implications for psychiatric nosology and research. *Shanghai Arch Psychiatry*. 2015;27(2):82–86. https://doi.org/10.11919/j.issn.1002-0829.215041.

25. Scheepers FE, Mul J, Boer F, Hoogendijk WJ. Psychosis as an evolutionary adaptive mechanism to changing environments. *Frontiers in Psychiatry*. 2018;9:237. https://doi.org/10.3389/fpsyt.2018.00237.

26. Upthegrove R, Marwaha S, Birchwood M. Depression and schizophrenia: cause, consequence, or transdiagnostic issue? *Schizophrenia Bulletin*. 2017;43(2):240–244. https://doi.org/10.1093/schbul/sbw097.

27. Kahn JP, Bombassaro T, Veras AB. Comorbid schizophrenia and panic anxiety: panic psychosis revisited. *Psychiatric Annals*. 2018;48(12):561–565. https://doi.org/10.3928/00485713-20181113-01.

28. Savitz AJ, Kahn TA, McGovern KE, Kahn JP. Carbon dioxide induction of panic anxiety in schizophrenia with auditory hallucinations. *Psychiatry Research*. 2011;189(1):38–42. https://doi.org/10.1016/j.psychres.2011.06.008.

29. Chan V. Schizophrenia and psychosis: Diagnosis, current research trends, and model treatment approaches with implications for transitional age youth. *Child and Adolescent Psychiatric Clinics of North America*. 2017;26(2):341–366. https://doi.org/10.1016/j.chc.2016.12.014.

30. Van Os J, Reininghaus U. Psychosis as a transdiagnostic and extended phenotype in the general population. *World Psychiatry*. 2016;15(2):118–124. https://doi.org/10.1002/wps.20310.

31. Catalan A, Simons CJP, Bustamante S, Olazabal N, Ruiz E, Artaza MG, et al. Data gathering bias: trait vulnerability to psychotic symptoms? *PLoS One*. 2015;10(8):e0135761.

32. Zalpuri I, Rothschild AJ. Does psychosis increase the risk of suicide in patients with major depression? A systematic review. *Journal of Affective Disorders*. 2016;198:23–31. https://doi.org/10.1016/j.jad.2016.03.035.

33. Rutigliano G, Valmaggia L, Landi P, Frascarelli M, Cappucciati M, Sear V, et al. Persistence or recurrence of non-psychotic comorbid mental disorders associated with 6-year poor functional outcomes in patients at ultra high risk for psychosis. *Journal of Affective Disorders*. 2016;203:101–110. https://doi.org/10.1016/j.jad.2016.05.053.

34. Fusar-Poli P, Yung AR, McGorry P, Van Os J. Lessons learned from the psychosis high-risk state: towards a general staging model of prodromal intervention. *Psychological Medicine*. 2014;44(1):17–24. https://doi.org/10.1017/S0033291713000184.

35. McGorry, P. D., Hartmann, J. A., Spooner, R., & Nelson, B. (2018). Beyond the "at risk mental state" concept: transitioning to transdiagnostic psychiatry. *World Psychiatry*, 17(2), 133–142. doi: https://doi.org/10.1002/wps.20514.

CHAPTER 2

Psychotogenesis

Nadia Rahman   Sulaima Daboul   Emeka Boka   Dolores Malaspina

Abstract

What are the underlying causes of psychosis? Why do certain members of the general population experience hallucinations but remain functional while other members enter the psychosis prodrome, and still others go on to experience full-fledged psychosis? In this chapter we will review the putative risk factors associated with psychosis and explore current theories on the pathogenesis of psychosis. We begin with a brief history of psychosis that reviews schizophrenia and related psychosis disorders. Next, we explore genetic risk factors and environmental exposures for psychosis. We conclude this chapter with an overview of current theories regarding the pathophysiology of psychosis and early predictors of psychosis.

KEYWORDS

Psychosis	Premorbid	Risk pathways	Schizophrenia	Schizoaffective
Cannabis	Paternal age			

Introduction

As described since ancient times, and by Hippocrates 2000 years ago, psychosis is a mental state characterized by impaired reality testing.[1] It is manifest as a constellation of symptoms, including false perceptions and fixed false beliefs, called "hallucinations" and "delusions," and through disturbed thinking evidenced by the use of language, including "loose associations," and frequently through bizarre motor activity and behavior. Schizophrenia is the best-known psychotic disorder, and many of the classic symptoms of psychosis were originally observed in patients who would currently be diagnosed as having schizophrenia.

Eugen Bleuler (1857–1939), the Swiss psychiatrist who coined the term "schizophrenia" (from the Greek *skhizein* "to split" and *phren* "mind"), considered psychotic symptoms to arise from a "break" (disconnection) between the neural systems subserving thought and emotion. He proposed that this schism produced observable phenomena, later referred to as the four A's, including autistic preoccupation, ambivalence, affect (flat), and associations (loose, which are characteristic of thought disorder). All of these, except ambivalence, continue to be key criteria for the diagnosis of schizophrenia in modern diagnostic procedures.[2] Kurt Schneider (1887–1967), a German psychiatrist, later compiled a core group of "hallmark" psychotic symptoms termed "first rank symptoms" (FRSs), which he proposed could distinguish schizophrenia from other psychotic disorders. These were the experiences of audible thoughts, hallucinations of two or more individuals arguing or conversing, voices that commented on the patient's actions, thought broadcasting, thought withdrawal or insertion, delusions of passivity, and delusional perception. But in more recent years, studies have shown that these are not specific to schizophrenia.[3]

While psychosis is a defining feature of schizophrenia spectrum disorders, it is a variable feature in conditions such as substance use, developmental, endocrine, and brain disorders and diseases.[4] Substance abuse including alcohol, amphetamines, hallucinogens, marijuana, and opioids can all cause isolated periods of psychosis. Substance-induced psychosis is diagnostically distinct from other psychotic disorders in that symptoms subside shortly after substance use, while psychotic symptoms in psychotic disorders continue and may be chronic.[5] Psychotic symptoms are also observed in other disorders, including bipolar disorder, depression with psychotic features, post-traumatic stress disorder and obsessive-compulsive disorder (OCD), some personality disorders, and in subclinical quantities in some persons without mental illness. It has also been proposed that there could be psychoses associated with anxiety disorders such as social anxiety, panic anxiety, and OCD.[6-9]

Psychosis has historically been split into two dichotomous categories: affective (including bipolar disorder and major depressive disorder with psychotic features) and non-affective psychosis (including schizophrenia and schizoaffective disorder). In recent years, the validity of the nosologic distinction between these two categories has been called into question and a transdiagnostic dimensional approach has been put forth as a more ecologically valid way of conceptualizing psychosis-related disorders. Research using factor analysis has shown that a general, transdiagnostic dimension that includes affective and non-affective symptoms in addition to five symptom dimensions (depression, mania, positive symptoms, negative symptoms, and disorganization) may better model the different forms of psychosis experienced by patients. This model is called the bifactor model.[10,11]

The central thesis of this book is that psychosis proneness may interact with certain comorbidities (including OCD, panic disorder, social anxiety, major depressive disorder, mania, substance abuse, and medical illnesses) and other factors (including environmental and genetic) to produce different forms of psychosis. In this chapter, we will discuss the pathogenesis of psychosis and factors related to its development. The terms "psychosis" and "schizophrenia" will be used somewhat interchangeably due to the fact that the bulk of the extant research focuses on schizophrenia. Presently, we will review psychosis as it is featured in schizophrenia and other psychosis-related disorders.

Psychosis in Schizophrenia

Characteristic symptoms for a diagnosis of schizophrenia include profound deficits in emotion and behavior, interfering with the expression of emotion and with motivation, often referred to as flat affect and avolition. As these are the absence of normal functions, they are called negative symptoms, distinguishing these from the active psychotic symptoms, conversely named the positive symptoms. The schizophrenia diagnosis also includes deterioration in functioning, a phenomena that typically occurs before the emergence of psychotic symptoms.[12] In the last century, it has become evident the positive and negative symptoms associated with schizophrenia are highly variable between individual patients.

This observation led to the concept of "the group of schizophrenias" by Bleuler,[13] but the differential determinants of etiology and optimum precision treatments for schizophrenia remain unclear. Most patients are initially affected in young adulthood; 50% go on to experience some disability throughout their lives, and an additional 25% never recover and require lifelong care.[14] The lifetime risk for schizophrenia is commonly reported to be approximately 1% and to be similar for men and women, with an earlier onset in males. However, recent epidemiologic reviews demonstrate a prominent geographic variation in incidence, with a fivefold variation around a median incidence of 15.2/100,000 persons (7.7–43.0/100,000), and more affected males than females (1.4:1).[15]

Distinguishing Psychotic Depression and Bipolar Disorder

Among persons with psychosis and deterioration, schizophrenia spectrum conditions are traditionally distinguished from mood-related psychosis, including bipolar and other affective disorders. However, the diagnostic boundary between the affective and non-affective (schizophrenia) psychoses is an active topic of debate. Emil Kraepelin (1856–1926) was the first to dichotomize affective and non-affective psychotic conditions. He provided the earliest rigorous descriptions of *dementia praecox* (now denoted as schizophrenia) and observed differences between these cases and those with manic-depressive insanity (now denoted as bipolar disorder) in the episodicity of their symptoms and long-term outcome. His idea was that these were dichotomous conditions with different underpinnings.[14] This was one of the earliest attempts to categorize mental illnesses based on observable behavioral phenomena. The separateness of these conditions, while still retained in separate chapters of the DSM-5, is challenged by diagnostic instability and overlap in their epidemiology, genetics, neuroanatomy, and neuropsychiatric finding.[12]

Schizoaffective Disorder

Psychosis can occur during an episode of depression or mania, or other psychiatric disease in which it is diagnosed as a component of the primary psychiatric condition. However, persons with schizophrenia can also experience mood episodes. Of course, as above, if the full mood syndrome is always present or treated during the psychotic episodes, the diagnosis is not schizophrenia. It has been more problematic to name a condition that includes periods of psychosis without any mood disturbance, of at least 2 weeks, with other periods of psychosis including full manic, mixed, or depressive episodes. When such mood syndromes occur, less than half of the total duration of all periods during which there are psychotic or residual symptoms, the DSM-5 diagnosis is schizophrenia and a separate mood diagnosis. If full mood syndromes have been present for more than half of the total duration of all psychotic plus residual periods (> 50%), which the clinician estimates, then the diagnosis is schizoaffective disorder, either depressed or bipolar.[12]

Psychosis in Community Samples

Notably, some members of the general population have odd experiences that verge on hallucinations or delusions, others enter the psychosis prodrome, and still others develop full-fledged psychosis.[16] Studies done in community samples indicate that psychotic-like experiences are not uncommon in the general population. Indeed, the incidence of psychotic symptoms occurring in the general population is approximately between 4.8% and 8.3% depending on the particular symptom being examined.[17] These psychotic-like symptoms may represent variations on normal personality traits or they may be forme frustes indicative of an underlying vulnerability to a psychotic disorder.

One theory posits that positive psychotic symptoms exist on a continuum, with full-fledged psychosis on one end and psychotic-like symptoms on the other end. Two models of continuity have been put forth: the quasi-dimensional model and the fully dimensional model.[18] The quasi-dimensional model theorizes that psychotic-like symptoms represent partial penetrance of psychosis, and those exhibiting such symptoms would be at an increased vulnerability for the development of a psychotic disorder. This model implies a discontinuity from the normal population. Paul Meehl supported this theory, coining the term "schizotaxia" to describe the symptomatic, cognitive, and behavioral vulnerabilities that are likely to eventuate in a diagnosis of schizophrenia. By contrast, the fully dimensional model of psychosis posits no discontinuity from a healthy population suggesting that psychotic-like symptoms are a feature of personality.[19]

Psychosis Prodrome

The criteria for the prodromal phase of psychosis is a period of functional deterioration before the onset of the full-blown active symptoms of psychosis. Individuals within this phase are considered to be at clinical high risk for a transition to psychosis. The diagnosis of clinical high risk is warranted when there is a presence of at least one of the following: (1) functional impairment (social and occupational) in the context of familial risk; (2) brief limited intermittent psychotic symptoms (BLIPS—an episode of severe psychotic symptoms, which resolves spontaneously within 1 week and occurred during the past 12 months); or (3) attenuated psychotic symptoms (APS).[20–22] According to the DSM-5, APS include perceptual disturbances (subthreshold hallucination), overvalued ideas (subthreshold delusions), and disorganized speech, all with relatively unimpaired reality testing.[12,18] Approximately 36% of clinical high-risk individuals will transition to first episode frank psychosis after 3 years, follow-up, with half of the transitions (18%) occurring after the first 6 months.[23]

Schizotypy

Schizotypy represents a latent and persisting set of social oddities, cognitive problems, and personality disturbances that can lead to an array of schizophrenia-related phenotypes. Unlike the prodromal state of psychosis, schizotypy is more enduring. These phenotypic outcomes can manifest as overt personality disorders (e.g., schizotypal personality disorder, schizoid personality disorder, paranoid personality disorder, and avoidant personality disorder) or as a more tenuous subclinical presentation (e.g., interpersonal aversiveness, perceptual aberrations, referential thinking, magical ideation).[24] Schizotypy can also manifest as non-psychotic endophenotypes invisible to the naked eye but detectable with applicable technologies. These endophenotypes include sustained attention deficits, eye-tracking dysfunction, working memory impairments, motor dysfunction, thought disorder (secondary cognitive slippage), and psychometric deviance (PAS).[25]

Schizoid and schizotypal personality disorders are both cluster A personality disorders that are characterized by odd or eccentric thinking and behavior. Although these disorders resemble schizophrenia, they are diagnostically distinct categories. Schizotypal personality disorder encompasses a pervasive pattern of social deficits that may include cognitive or perceptual distortions, eccentric behavior, and unusual thinking. These symptoms may resemble positive schizophrenia symptoms. Individuals with schizoid personality disorder tend to prefer being alone, have difficulty understanding social cues, and may lack motivation in their professional lives. These symptoms may resemble negative schizophrenia symptoms. While many of the cluster A personality disorder symptoms overlap with schizophrenia symptoms, they never progress into full-fledged hallucinations or delusions. For example, while a person with schizotypal personality disorder may believe that the news anchor that night was broadcasting a story about their own life, when they are confronted with evidence contradicting their belief, they are able to modify their beliefs, whereas an individual with schizophrenia will not be dissuaded that the news story was not about them.[12]

While genetic claims regarding schizoid personality disorder's link to schizophrenia remain inconclusive, there is compelling evidence demonstrating the genetic overlap between schizotypal personality disorder and schizophrenia. Indeed, 40% of those who receive a diagnosis of schizotypal personality disorder progress to some psychotic disorder within the span of 2 years. The last decade has brought a burgeoning body of genetic research, including twin studies and linkage studies, that highlight the overlap between schizotypal personality traits and schizophrenia.[26]

The outcome and clinical course of schizotypy are still not fully understood. Many individuals with the phenomenon will never develop full-blown, active symptoms of psychosis (this is also true of individuals with prodromal psychotic symptoms). As conceived by Lenzenweger, individuals at the prodromal phase of psychosis who do not transition to frank psychosis are harboring schizotypy and will subsequently demonstrate a level of impairment in personality throughout a life span.[24] A recent study, however, does suggest premorbid schizotypy as an independent risk factor for transition to psychosis in the clinical high risk. In their study, Kotlicka-Antczak et al.[21] demonstrated that premorbid schizotypy, as elicited through mothers of individuals at clinical high risk, might be time-independently associated with the transition to psychosis. This finding was much more notable in clinical high-risk individuals with high levels of premorbid negative schizotypy (social isolation, restricted affect, and social anxiety/suspiciousness). It is also of importance to note that this positive correlation to psychosis transition was not only evident in clinical high risk with premorbid core schizotypy but was significantly present with antisocial aspects of schizotypal expression as well.[21]

Risk Factors for Psychosis

Only a small proportion of the population-attributable risk for schizophrenia can be explained by our current knowledge. Interactions between genes and exposures, particularly in certain developmental windows, will almost certainly be important. Increasingly, it is clear that gene-environment interactions must be considered for illness risk, with changes in gene expression as the likely mechanism.[27] Data that support models of interaction between genetic vulnerability and the environment result from adoption studies. For adopted-away children of mothers with schizophrenia, adversity and poor family functioning in the adoptive home increase the risk of schizophrenia; however, no such effect is seen for adopted-away children of healthy mothers.[28] In an Israeli study, children of mothers with schizophrenia had a higher risk of developing the illness themselves if raised in a kibbutz instead of a family home; again, this effect was not seen for children without genetic risk.[29] Among the interesting findings of gene-environment interaction for schizophrenia was the observed interaction of a specific allele of a susceptibility gene, val-COMT, with an exposure (specifically cannabis abuse), in increasing schizophrenia risk.[30] While val-COMT's primary role is the enzymatic degradation of adrenaline, noradrenaline, and dopamine, it is also thought to play a secondary role in the expression of both anxiety and depression.[31] Whether or not the observation of the gene-environment interaction with val-COMT stands up, it is a useful approach and may help inform future studies examining gene-environment interaction.

Global Genetic Risk Factors

Evidence from family, twin, and adoption studies suggests that the cause of schizophrenia is, at least in part, inherited. First-degree relatives of schizophrenic probands have an increased risk of schizophrenia, with estimated risk rates of 6% for parents, 10% for siblings, 13% for children with one affected parent, and 45% for children with two affected parents.[32] Identical twins have a concordance rate of 53%, whereas fraternal twins have a concordance rate of 15%.[33] The disparity in these rates suggest that 60% to 90% of schizophrenia liability can be attributed to genes.[34,35] Of interest, offspring of affected and unaffected (discordant) monozygotic twins have equal risk for schizophrenia (about 16%–18%), consistent with either incomplete penetrance and/or gene-environment interaction. Adoption studies also support inheritance of schizophrenia liability,[36,37] though cannot discriminate if such effects are genetic or environmental (in utero) if mothers are the parent of comparison. When fathers are the parent in common (paternal half-siblings), however, the same increased risk in biological (vs. adopted) relatives holds.[38] Adoption studies also provide evidence for gene-environment interaction, as adopted-away children of biologic mothers with schizophrenia are even more likely to develop schizophrenia if they are raised in an adverse environment.[28,39]

The consistent evidence of inherited vulnerability revealed by a century of family twin and adoption studies of schizophrenia risk encouraged genetic research in schizophrenia. Dozens of candidate studies, genetic linkage, and association research studies were published, but not replicated. It is only with the advent of the hypothesis-independent genome-wide association studies (GWAS) approach that the Psychiatric Genetics Consortium uncovered scores of common loci that are significantly associated with schizophrenia, with increasing numbers of loci identified as sample sizes increased. These studies highlight the importance of immune factors, calcium signaling, N-methyl-D-aspartic acid (NMDA) glutamatergic function, and synaptic elements for schizophrenia risk, but the majority of common gene findings are not specific for schizophrenia. Notably the genetic risk architecture for schizophrenia also includes copy number variants (CNV), estimated to account for 5% of cases.[40] These intermediate-sized gene variants can influence the expression and function of many genes,[41] with certain very rare CNVs associated with a manifold increase in the risk for schizophrenia.[42]

Other Family Risk Factors

LATE PATERNAL AGE

The genetic architecture of schizophrenia particularly includes many novel or rare versions of genes. The intriguing notion that schizophrenia can result from de novo genetic events in the paternal germ line was first suggested by Malaspina et al.[43] to explain the robust relationship of paternal age on the risk for schizophrenia.[44] Since then, multiple studies in diverse populations have replicated the paternal age effect.[45,46] In the Malaspina cohort, paternal age, overall, explained over 25% of the risk for schizophrenia. Comparably, in Sweden, Rasmussen estimated that 15% of cases were attributable to paternal age greater than 30 years. The paternal age effect appears to be restricted to cases without a family history of psychosis.[46,47] Sipos found that paternal age was unrelated to the risk for familial cases, whereas the offspring of the oldest fathers showed a 5.5-fold increased risk for sporadic (nonfamilial) schizophrenia. The epidemiologic evidence is convincing. There is a "dosage effect" of increasing paternal age on the relative risk for schizophrenia, and each cohort study has shown an approximately tripling of risk for the offspring of the oldest fathers (> 45–55 years). The studies have employed prospective exposure data and used validated psychiatric diagnoses, and they have together controlled for potential confounding factors such as family history, maternal age, parental education and social ability, social class, birth order, birth weight, and birth complications. Furthermore, the studies show a specificity of late paternal age on the risk for schizophrenia versus other psychiatric disorders, which is not the case for any other schizophrenia risk factor, including most of the susceptibility alleles (vide infra). Furthermore, there is some evidence that sporadic (paternal age related) schizophrenia may be a particular variant of the disease from familial cases.[48] The relationship between advanced paternal age and schizophrenia risk has been attributed to chromosomal aberrations and changes in the aging germline. This same mechanism was used to explain other chromosomal and neoplastic diseases in which the advanced paternal age was a major risk factor.

EARLY MATERNAL AGE

Young maternal age at birth is associated with an increased offspring risk for schizophrenia.[49,50] However, the basis of this relationship has many possible explanations. Leading hypotheses include impulsive behavior by young women who carry schizophrenia susceptibility genes that are then transmitted to the early-born offspring,[15,51] less skilled parenting by immature women,[52] and a newer version of the "schizophrenogenic mother" hypothesis.[53,54] Others suggested prenatal effects wherein maternal resources are held back from the fetus in earlier pregnancies to be available at later ones.[55,56]

SHORT DURATION OF MARRIAGE

Shorter duration of marriage has been associated with increased risk of schizophrenia in off-spring. This risk is independent of any parental psychiatric disorder and/or paternal age at birth. A recent study based on data from Jerusalem Perinatal Cohort Schizophrenia Study (JPSS), which documented births in Jerusalem from 1964 to 1976,[50] demonstrated a 50% increase in risk for schizophrenia in offspring of parents with less than 2 years of marriage and a 30% increase in risk in offspring of parents with 2 to 4 years of marriage.[49] Moreover, this risk corresponds with obstetric findings showing increased risk of preeclampsia in shorter duration of marriage in a similar way, due to maternal immune intolerance to paternal antigens.[15,57] Therefore, duration of marriage is a modifiable risk factor with longer durations of marriage that corresponds with longer maternal exposure to paternal antigens. This lowers the maternal immune intolerance and promotes healthier outcomes.

BIRTH ORDER

A certain birth order constitutes a risk factor for psychosis in general and schizophrenia specifically.[49,50] This risk was highest among first-born males and last-born females.[15] This risk is independent of any covariables such as desire of pregnancy, perinatal effects, maternal age at delivery, maternal schizophrenic status, and number of siblings. Underlying causes can be related to biological components and/or different stressors within a specific birth order. In addition, the risk related to shorter duration of marriage may account for this excess risk in firstborn offspring compared to other siblings, as parents certainly have shorter sexual cohabitation at first births.

Environmental Exposures

Presently, we will review the putative environmental exposures associated with schizophrenia risk. These risk factors include prenatal adversity, childhood trauma, childhood infections, traumatic brain injury (TBI), discrimination, immigration status, urban birth, and cannabis use. It is important to note that most exposures have small effects, with typical odds ratios or risk ratios of approximately 2. Questions of causation remain about some premorbid or prodromal syndromes that could increase risk of exposure (i.e., to head injury or drug use).

PRENATAL ADVERSITY

It has been well established that obstetric complications carry an increased risk for schizophrenia in offspring. Three common complications that show up often in most literature are prenatal complications, fetal growth retardation, and perinatal hypoxia.[58] Therefore, the prenatal exposure to any kind of stressor activates proinflammatory cytokines that cause changes in the brain development pathway. These changes underline the pathophysiology of these neuropsychiatric disorders. For example, Sorensen and colleagues found that prenatal analgesics exposure in the second trimester is associated with an increased risk of schizophrenia. This was true even after confounding for any possible factors. There is a higher prevalence of schizophrenia among individuals born in the winter and early spring,[59] consistent with associations of maternal infections during pregnancy with schizophrenia risk (up to sevenfold), including rubella,[60] influenza,[61] and toxoplasmosis.[62] Postnatal infections (especially neonatal coxsackie B meningitis) are also associated with later schizophrenia.[63] Other intrauterine and obstetric risk factors besides infection associated with later schizophrenia include pre-eclampsia, low birthweight, hypoxic events,[64] maternal cigarette smoking,[65] Rh incompatibility,[66] maternal stress,[67] and exposure to famine or malnutrition early in gestation (i.e., the Dutch Hunger Winter of 1944–1945).[68,69]

CHILDHOOD TRAUMA

Childhood trauma is associated with several negative mental health outcomes. Experiencing psychotic episodes that transform to psychosis is a consistently found outcome. This includes all types of trauma, including sexual, emotional, and physical abuse. Moreover, this association was found to be dose-dependent in several studies that were based on the adverse childhood experience study. Therefore, there is a positively graded relationship between the increasing childhood trauma and the negative mental health outcome.[70–72] Bebbington and colleagues found that the strongest association was the one between psychosis and child sexual trauma.[73] In addition, Kelleher and colleagues concluded that discontinuance of the traumatic events lowers the psychotic experiences prevalence.[74]

CHILDHOOD INFECTIONS

Childhood infections have been found to carry an increased risk for psychotic disorders later in life. A number of researchers examined the effect of the 1957 influenza epidemic and found an increased risk for schizophrenia was associated with infections in the second trimester.[70–74] In addition, Brown and colleagues found an increased risk for schizophrenia spectrum disorders was associated with some respiratory infections and rubella infection.[75,76] Moreover, Suvisaari and colleagues found an association between second-trimester polio virus infection and risk of developing schizophrenia later in life.[77]

TRAUMATIC BRAIN INJURY

Incidence of post-TBI psychotic disorders has been studied for several years. However, this incidence rate ranged from 0.1% to 9.8%, and there were several limitations to these studies, including the retrospective design and the difference between the old and the new diagnostic criteria.[78]

DISCRIMINATION

Recent studies have demonstrated that individuals at clinical high risk significantly report more perceived discrimination in contrast to controls.[79] This finding is independent of general suspiciousness or other APS. In these individuals, perceived discrimination was a positive predictive indicator of future transition to frank psychosis.

IMMIGRATION STATUS

Furthermore, there exists an increased incidence of schizophrenia among immigrants versus non-immigrants, especially in individuals immigrating from predominantly dark-skinned countries to predominantly white-skinned countries. These findings have also been demonstrated in children of these immigrants as well. According to Egerton and colleagues, clinical high-risk immigrants residing in the United Kingdom and Canada demonstrated this positive correlation to psychosis. Studies indicate a significant elevation in striatal dopamine function among immigrants living in the United Kingdom and Canada compared to non-immigrants.[80] Immigration is associated with somewhat higher risk, compared with other exposures, as migration from poor countries to wealthy countries is associated with a 3- to 10-fold increase in schizophrenia risk, compared with both the host country and the country of origin (reviewed in Jones and Cannon).[35] This effect is greater for second-generation than for first-generation migrants, arguing against selective migration of at-risk individuals. It is not clear whether this finding reflects the effect of urbanization, stress, racism, or exposure to some new infectious or other environmental agent.

URBAN BIRTH

Urban dwelling is a well-established risk factor for developing psychosis (see the section on population-based risk factors above). This phenomenon, however, has not been sufficiently researched among clinical high-risk individuals. This correlation, or lack thereof, remains unknown and an area of great interest.[81]

CANNABIS USE

Cannabis is a very commonly used drug and is associated with the development of psychosis, especially with the use of high-potency forms (see the section on population-based risk factors above). Studies demonstrate that clinical high-risk individuals significantly use cannabis twice as much when compared to healthy controls and are also five times more likely to suffer from cannabis use disorder.[82] There is a significant increase in symptom severity in users, including an increase in thought content and suspiciousness. The lifetime prevalence of cannabis use of clinical high-risk individuals is 53%, which is quite similar to the prevalence of cannabis use in first-episode psychosis[82] and significantly lower than in healthy controls. Although there is increased use of cannabis in clinical high-risk individuals, that alone does not seem to predict transition to psychosis. As demonstrated by Kraan and colleagues, cannabis use in clinical high-risk individuals and transition to psychosis seems to be dose dependent. Individuals that meet the criteria for cannabis abuse or cannabis dependence are positive predictors of transition to psychosis.[83]

Pathophysiology of Psychosis

NEUROTRANSMITTER ABNORMALITIES

Dopamine

Dopamine is a neurotransmitter that plays a major role in our brains' reward and motivation pathway; it promotes pleasure-seeking behaviors. Converging research has found deficient dopamine release in the prefrontal cortex in schizophrenia. This finding has emerged from evidence implicating deficient dopamine release in the impaired working memory seen in schizophrenic patients.[84] Other research has linked excessive subcortical transmission of dopamine to the severity of psychotic symptoms in schizophrenia[85] and to the risk of conversion to psychosis among persons considered to be at high risk for the disease.[86] What's more, many antipsychotics that operate as antagonists for D2 receptor functioning are used to treat the non-affective and affective symptoms of psychosis.[87] More research needs to be done to elucidate the relationship between dopamine signaling and schizophrenia.

Glutamate and Gamma-Aminobutyric Acid

Previous research has implicated dysfunction of glutamate signaling through NMDA receptors in the pathophysiology of schizophrenia. NMDA receptors play a role in synaptic plasticity and memory function in the brain and glutamate is a nonessential amino acid that is the brain's main excitatory neurotransmitter, coordinating the cortex, limbic system, and thalamus (brain regions that have been implicated in schizophrenia). Glutamate also acts as the precursor for gamma-aminobutyric acid (GABA), the brain's main inhibitory neurotransmitter. Blockage of the NMDA receptor by dissociative anesthetics such as phenylcyclohexyl piperidine produces similar psychotic, negative, and cognitive symptoms to those seen in schizophrenia. Enhancing agents for NMDA receptor functioning have demonstrably improved cognitive functioning and negative symptoms in schizophrenic patients being treated with typical antipsychotics.[88]

Deficient GABAergic signaling has also been associated with schizophrenia.[11] An inclusive model, devised by Lodge and Grace[89] posits that dysregulation of the subcortical dopamine system produces psychotic symptoms. However, this may be a consequence of hippocampal pathology acting through failures in inhibitory GABAergic interneurons and/or excessive glutaminergic activity.[89] Indeed, hippocampal hyperactivity is correlated with psychotic symptoms.[86]

OVER-PRUNING OF SYNAPSES

The development of new neurons and the formation of synapses begins in the preliminary stages of embryonic development and continues at an elevated rate until about 2 years of age. At that point, individuals possess many more neurons and synaptic connections than are functionally necessary. Synaptic pruning is the process by which extraneous neurons and synaptic connections are weeded out for the purpose of optimizing neuronal transmissions.[90] Pruning occurs very quickly between the ages of 2 and 10, and occurs in the cerebral cortex throughout adolescence at a reduced rate. While it was previously thought that the process of synaptic pruning is terminated after adolescence, recent findings demonstrate that pruning continues throughout the third decade of life and stabilizes around the age of 30.[91]

In recent years, post-mortem analysis of cortical tissue from patients with schizophrenia has demonstrated a marked reduction in synaptic density, suggesting over-pruning of synapses in this population. Specifically, these studies show increased packing of neuron cell bodies, with decreased white matter where the synapses connect, specifically dendritic branches and their spines,[92,93] and abnormal expression of a host of synaptic proteins and their corresponding messenger RNA.[93–96] Given significant removal of synapses in the cerebral cortex during late adolescence and early adulthood, the same period during which the onset of schizophrenia typically occurs, it has been hypothesized that excessive pruning of synapses contributes to the reduction in synaptic density observed in patients with schizophrenia.[97]

IMMUNE ACTIVATION OF SYNAPSES

More recent studies implicate abnormal immune activation as a key pathology for schizophrenia with complement-mediated neuronal cell death leading to "synaptic pruning," the excessive loss of neurons observed for psychosis prone individuals during late adolescent development.[98]

HYPOFRONTALITY

The frontal lobe is a brain region responsible for the planning of complex behavior, decision making, personality expression, and the processing of social behavior. There is a long history of research implicating both thinning and reduced functioning in the frontal cortex with schizophrenia. Thinning of the frontal cortex appears to be present at the onset of psychosis, but the extent of this thinning effect is unrelated to symptom severity or functioning level.[99] This gives us some insight into causality, as thinning of the frontal cortex is unlikely to be caused by psychosis or antipsychotic medicine. Decreased metacognitive insight is associated with thinning of the frontal lobe. Moreover, cognitive dysfunction apparent in schizophrenia and related mood disorders is theorized to be caused by reduced inferior frontal lobe volume.[100] Taken together, these research findings suggest that hypofrontality may play a role in the social and cognitive impairment seen in schizophrenia.

GENETIC MARKERS

A robust body of research—including family, twin, and adoption studies studies—has demonstrated the heritability of schizophrenia.[26] The lifetime risk of schizophrenia is 1% for the general population and, by contrast, this risk rises to over 40% in monozygotic twins of people with schizophrenia.[101]

After the early promising results of candidate gene studies and linkage analyses in patients with schizophrenia and their families failed replication attempts, knowledge about the genetic basis of schizophrenia was finally advanced through the development of Genome Wide Association Studies. This approach identifies the risk for a disease that is attributable to common variations at individual single nucleotides in very large samples of cases. Of interest to this discussion, a genetic relationship between the genetic profile for schizophrenia was demonstrated to positive, cognitive, and negative psychotic-like experiences in adolescence, especially to cognitive disorganization, anhedonia, and psychotic-like symptoms. Taken together, these findings lend support for the theory that the schizophrenia and schizotypy may have the same biological underpinnings.

Predictors of Psychosis

COGNITION

According to several longitudinal studies reviewed by Addington et al., apparent deficits in cognitive function are suggestive of transition to psychosis. However, there is a lack of consensus on the exact cognitive domains involved. Several studies indicate that the most commonly observed cognitive impairments in clinical high-risk individuals who will transition to frank psychosis versus those who will not include verbal memory and processing speed, verbal learning, verbal fluency, working memory, and attention.[79] Although most clinical high-risk individuals present with a social cognitive deficit, this impairment does not draw a parallel with the transition to psychosis after controlling for IQ, education, and baseline symptoms as illustrated in a meta-analysis reviewed by Addington et al.

FUNCTIONAL IMPAIRMENT

Functional impairment is a well-established criterion for psychotic disorders such as schizophrenia. This functional impairment, if present in individuals at clinical high risk, has a strong positive correlation in predicting transition to psychosis. Addington et al., as illustrated in their meta-analysis review of several longitudinal studies, reported significantly lower baseline global functioning (using the Global Assessment of Functioning Scale) in clinical high-risk individuals who transitioned to frank psychosis versus those who did not. Impairment in premorbid functioning (before the onset of the prodromal phase of psychosis) is independently associated with the transition to frank psychosis only at the late adolescent stage (16–18 years).[102] In clinical high-risk individuals, further classification into two domains reveals that poor social functioning is predictive of transitioning, while poor role functioning is not predictive of transitioning to psychosis.[79]

NEUROIMAGING

Multiple studies by Fusar-Poli et al.,[23] Cannon et al.,[34] and Chung et al., as reviewed by Addington and colleagues, indicate that structural brain changes in the clinical high risk are associated with the transition to psychosis. There are two distinct types of brain changes evident based on age groups. Clinical high-risk individuals between age 12 and 17 years who transition to psychosis demonstrated variations between brain age and chronologic age, which was overestimated. Furthermore, clinical high-risk individuals age 18 and above that transition to psychosis were found to have an increased rate of gray matter loss, mainly in the frontal lobes.[79] These structural changes were significant when compared to non-transitioning clinical high-risk individuals. Other studies suggest similar findings throughout the brain, including all four lobes as well as the cerebellum.[103,104] Most recent studies indicate functional abnormalities in both the medial (specifically the hippocampus) and lateral temporal lobes in clinical high-risk cohorts who transitioned to psychosis.[20] Other brain structural abnormalities found in clinical high-risk individuals predictive of transition to psychosis include malformations in gyrification,[105] cerebello-thalamic-cortical circuit hyperconnectivity at baseline in functional MRI (fMRI), and thalamic dysconnectivity.[106]

NEUROPHYSIOLOGY

Events-related potentials (ERPSs) are associated with the development of psychosis in the clinical high risk, namely sensory gating, mismatch negativity (MMN), and P300.[107] However, according to a meta-analysis by Bodatsch et al., MMN has demonstrated the most convincing evidence as an individual predictor of transition in the clinical high risk. A more recent and highly powered study by Tang et al. demonstrated a lower fronto-central P300 novel amplitude as well as minimally lower P300 oddball amplitude in clinical high-risk individuals who transitioned to psychosis after a 12-month follow-up.[108] Other studies as reviewed by Addington et al. suggest that changes in current source density in the beta and gamma band are predictive of transition, most notably in the left superior temporal gyrus, the left inferior parietal lobule, and the precuneus.[79]

OTHER BIOMARKERS

There are very few studies and inconclusive evidence that specific blood biomarkers are directly associated with the transition to psychosis. Early findings suggest the possibility of certain baseline inflammatory markers, oxidative stress, and dysregulation of the hypothalamic-pituitary axis.[79]

ENDOPHENOTYPES

Increased familial risk exists not only for schizophrenia but also for its spectrum disorders, such as schizotypal, paranoid, and schizoid personality disorder.[109,110] Some studies have focused on examining putative "endophenotypes" or "intermediate phenotypes" of putative genetic vulnerability for schizophrenia. These measures are thought to lie along the pathway between vulnerability and disease, including measures of psychophysiology, neuroimaging and electrophysiology. By definition, enndophenotypes are significantly more prevalent in cases than controls, are heritable and trait-like, and are also found also in family members without the disease. They are more objectively defined than illness status and can be studied in animal models to delineate pathophysiology. Promising candidate endophenotypes include aberrant smooth-pursuit eye movement,[111] N-acetyl aspartate concentrations in the hippocampus,[112] abnormal hippocampal morphology,[113] the P50 gating deficit[114] and abnormalities in working memory.[115]

Data from a recent large collaborative study examining endophenotypes and single nucleotide variants in schizophrenia (COGS) identified anti-saccades in eye movements, Continuous Performance Test-Identical Pairs 3-digit version scores, California Verbal Learning Test, and emotion identification as relevant endophenotypes that were over 80% accurate in identifying persons with schizophrenia. Nonetheless, the subset of endophenotypes was not equal to the clinical diagnosis in identifying the disease,[116] and thus unlikely to be of use in predicting who would develop the disease from general population or clinical samples. New findings show that neurons secrete exosomes or microvesicles that carry DNA and RNA molecules,[117] and are able to cross the brain-blood barrier (BBB) into the blood and cerebrospinal fluid (CSF).[118] They may prove to be useful for the diagnosis of schizophrenia vulnerability.

Premorbid Abnormalities Support Developmental Origins

Many types of premorbid deviations can be found at each age in some portion of subjects, including minor physical abnormalities, soft neurologic signs, delayed and suboptimal motor and language, social interest and capacity, and neurocognition. It was, indeed, nearly a half century ago that Fish and colleagues (1977) coined the phrase "pan-developmental retardation," to refer to the widespread subtle abnormalities in multiple domains, observed in children who later developed schizophrenia, including motor, sensory, cognitive, and cerebellar function.[119]

In line with models of psychotogenesis, many studies confirm the presence of early and subtle abnormalities in at-risk children, such as compromised psychomotor performance, and cognitive and motor dysfunction by age 10.[120,121] An innovative blinded review of home videos showed that raters could accurately identify which children would later develop schizophrenia, based on motor skills.[122] Other precursors of schizophrenia (albeit nonspecific) include delays in developmental milestones (i.e., walking and talking), more isolated play at ages 4 and 6, speech problems and clumsiness at ages 7 and 11, and poor school performance and social anxiety during the teen years.[123] Global attentional dysfunction may be a biobehavioral marker for genetic liability to schizophrenia, as attentional deficits exist in nearly half of all schizophrenia patients, and in the offspring of parents with schizophrenia.[57,124] Abnormal social behavior also may be another nonspecific indicator of risk for schizophrenia, i.e., trouble making friends, disciplinary problems, and unusual behavior in childhood and adolescence.[125] Early symptoms of premorbid anxiety disorders could also help explain abnormal social behavior seen in schizophrenia.[126]

Later Insults Associated with Schizophrenia

Early trauma has consistently been linked to the development of psychosis-related disorders. One study found that people who are victims of child abuse are three times more likely to develop psychosis than their counterparts who had never been abused.[127] Early trauma has also been associated with an earlier onset of schizophrenia, greater symptom severity, and the need for more aggressive treatment.[128,129] There is also evidence, however, that patients are not "doomed from the womb" and that a number of postnatal exposures may be associated with the risk for schizophrenia, including TBI[43] and the use of drugs, such as cannabis.[130] For some or many cases, there is evidence that progressive deterioration occurs in adulthood, so that any developmental lesion affects neural function across adulthood as well as in early stages. Evidence that neural damage may be ongoing is clearly demonstrated by changes beyond the onset of illness[131]: for example, the superior temporal gyrus decreases in volume after onset of first psychosis.[132]

While earlier family, twin, and adoption studies pointed to a likely pattern of heritability in schizophrenia, the last decade has been marked by significant advances in our understanding of the genetic underpinnings of schizophrenia, including the identification of specific genes and chromosomal regions likely implicated in the pathogenesis of schizophrenia. While such research has pointed to a likely genetic predisposition to schizophrenia, converging evidence from the last decade has also highlighted the role environmental factors that influence psychotogenesis, including early childhood experiences, drug use, identity, and physical environment. In addition to environmental factors, accompanying comorbidities may also help determine endophenotype. Comorbidity subtypes of particular interest—panic disorder, social anxiety disorder, melancholic depression, atypical depression, and OCD—are all conditions that frequently occur alongside psychosis.[9] Although not formally demonstrated, these comorbidity subtypes may correspond with the five specific factors seen in the bifactor model of psychosis (see introduction): positive symptoms, negative symptoms, depression, mania, and disorganization.[10,11] These comorbidity subtypes and the bifactor model will be explored further in subsequent chapters.

References

1. Sedivec V. Mental disorders in the writings of Hippocrates. *Cesk Psychiatr.* 1989;85:270–273.
2. Ashok AH, Baugh J, Yeragani VK. Paul Eugen Bleuler and the origin of the term schizophrenia (SCHIZOPRENIEGRUPPE). *Indian J Psychiatry.* 2012;54:95–96. https://doi.org/10.4103/0019-5545.94660.
3. Marneros A, Rohde A, Deister A, et al. Kurt Schneider's schizophrenia—the picture of schizophrenia in a Schneider-oriented university clinic. *Jpn J Psychiatry Neurol.* 1987;41:171–178.
4. Arciniegas DB. Psychosis. *Continuum (Minneap Minn).* 2015;21:715–736. https://doi.org/10.1212/01.CON.0000466662.89908.e7.
5. Kuzenko N, Sareen J, Beesdo-Baum K, et al. Associations between use of cocaine, amphetamines, or psychedelics and psychotic symptoms in a community sample. *Acta Psychiatr Scand.* 2011;123:466–474. https://doi.org/10.1111/j.1600-0447.2010.01633.x.
6. Galynker I, Ieronimo C, Perez-Acquino A, et al. Panic attacks with psychotic features. *J Clin Psychiatry.* 1996;57:402–406.
7. Rodriguez P, Holowka DW, Marx BP. Assessment of posttraumatic stress disorder-related functional impairment: a review. *J Rehabil Res Dev.* 2012;49:649–665.
8. Veras AB, do-Nascimento JS, Rodrigues RL, et al. Psychotic symptoms in social anxiety disorder patients: report of three cases. *Int Arch Med.* 2011;4:12. doi: https://doi.org/10.1186/1755-7682-4-12.
9. Kahn JP. *Angst: Origins of Anxiety and Depression.* New York: Oxford University Press; 2013.
10. Anderson AE, Marder S, Reise SP, et al. Bifactor modeling of the positive and negative syndrome scale: generalized psychosis spans schizoaffective, bipolar, and schizophrenia diagnoses. *Schizophr Bull.* 2018;44:1204–1216. https://doi.org/10.1093/schbul/sbx163.
11. Quattrone D, Di Forti M, Gayer-Anderson C, et al. Transdiagnostic dimensions of psychopathology at first episode psychosis: findings from the multinational EU-GEI study. *Psychol Med.* 2019;49:1378–1391. https://doi.org/10.1017/S0033291718002131.
12. American Psychiatric Association. *Diagnostic and statistical manual of mental disorders.* 5th ed. Washington, DC: Author; 2013.
13. Bleuler E. Dementia praecox or the group of schizophrenias. *JAMA.* 1951;145:685. https://doi.org/10.1001/jama.1951.02920270079043.
14. Hoff P. Eugen Bleuler's concept of schizophrenia and its relevance to present-day psychiatry. *Neuropsychobiology.* 2012;66:6–13. https://doi.org/10.1159/000337174.
15. McGrath J, Saha S, Chant D, et al. Schizophrenia: a concise overview of incidence, prevalence, and mortality. *Epidemiol Rev.* 2008;30:67–76. https://doi.org/10.1093/epirev/mxn001.
16. Broome MR, Woolley JB, Tabraham P, et al. What causes the onset of psychosis? *Schizophr Res.* 2005;79:23–34. https://doi.org/10.1016/j.schres.2005.02.007.
17. Nuevo R, Chatterji S, Verdes E, et al. The continuum of psychotic symptoms in the general population: a cross-national study. *Schizophr Bull.* 2012;38:475–485. https://doi.org/10.1093/schbul/sbq099.
18. Yung AR, Nelson B, Baker K, et al. Psychotic-like experiences in a community sample of adolescents: implications for the continuum model of psychosis and prediction of schizophrenia. *Aust NZ J Psychiatry.* 2009;43:118–128. https://doi.org/10.1080/00048670802607188.
19. Faraone SV, Green AI, Seidman LJ, et al. "Schizotaxia": clinical implications and new directions for research. *Schizophr Bull.* 2001;27:1–18. https://doi.org/10.1093/oxfordjournals.schbul.a006849.
20. Allen P, Moore H, Corcoran CM, et al. Emerging temporal lobe dysfunction in people at clinical high risk for psychosis. *Front Psychiatry.* 2019;10:298. https://doi.org/10.3389/fpsyt.2019.00298.
21. Kotlicka-Antczak M, Karbownik MS, Pawelczyk A, et al. A developmentally-stable pattern of premorbid schizoid-schizotypal features predicts psychotic transition from the clinical high-risk for psychosis state. *Compr Psychiatry.* 2019;90:95–101. https://doi.org/10.1016/j.comppsych.2019.02.003.
22. Yung AR, Yuen HP, McGorry PD, et al. Mapping the onset of psychosis: the Comprehensive Assessment of At-Risk Mental States. *Aust NZ J Psychiatry.* 2005;39:964–971. https://doi.org/10.1080/j.1440-1614.2005.01714.x.
23. Fusar-Poli P, Bonoldi I, Yung AR, et al. Predicting psychosis: meta-analysis of transition outcomes in individuals at high clinical risk. *Arch Gen Psychiatry.* 2012;69:220–229. https://doi.org/10.1001/archgenpsychiatry.2011.1472.
24. Lenzenweger MF. Schizotypy, schizotypic psychopathology and schizophrenia. *World Psychiatry.* 2018;17:25–26. https://doi.org/10.1002/wps.20479.

25. Lenzenweger MF, Lane MC, Loranger AW, et al. DSM-IV personality disorders in the National Comorbidity Survey Replication. *Biol Psychiatry*. 2007;62:553–564. https://doi.org/10.1016/j.biopsych.2006.09.019.

26. Pain O, Dudbridge F, Cardno AG, Freeman D, Lu Y, Lundstrom S, Lichtenstein P, Ronald A. Genome-wide analysis of adolescent psychotic-like experiences shows genetic overlap with psychiatric disorders. *American journal of medical genetics. Part B, Neuropsychiatric genetics : the official publication of the International Society of Psychiatric Genetics*. 2018;177(4):416–425. https://doi.org/10.1002/ajmg.b.32630.

27. Insel TR, Quirion R. Psychiatry as a clinical neuroscience discipline. *JAMA*. 2005;294:2221–2224. https://doi.org/10.1001/jama.294.17.2221.

28. Tienari P. Interaction between genetic vulnerability and family environment: the Finnish adoptive family study of schizophrenia. *Acta Psychiatr Scand*. 1991;84:460–465.

29. Mirsky AF, Yardley SL, Jones BP, et al. Analysis of the attention deficit in schizophrenia: a study of patients and their relatives in Ireland. *J Psychiatr Res*. 1995;29:23–42.

30. Caspi A, Moffitt TE, Cannon M, et al. Moderation of the effect of adolescent-onset cannabis use on adult psychosis by a functional polymorphism in the catechol-O-methyltransferase gene: longitudinal evidence of a gene X environment interaction. *Biol Psychiatry*. 2005;57:1117–1127. https://doi.org/10.1016/j.biopsych.2005.01.026.

31. Hoth KF, Paul RH, Williams LM, et al. Associations between the COMT Val/Met polymorphism, early life stress, and personality among healthy adults. *Neuropsychiatr Dis Treat*. 2006;2:219–225. https://doi.org/10.2147/nedt.2006.2.2.219.

32. Gottesman II, Bertelsen A. Confirming unexpressed genotypes for schizophrenia. Risks in the offspring of Fischer's Danish identical and fraternal discordant twins. *Arch Gen Psychiatry*. 1989;46:867–872. https://doi.org/10.1001/archpsyc.1989.01810100009002.

33. Mohindra KS, Haddad S, Narayana D. Women's health in a rural community in Kerala, India: do caste and socioeconomic position matter? *J Epidemiol Community Health*. 2006;60:1020–1026. https://doi.org/10.1136/jech.2006.047647.

34. Cannon TD, Kaprio J, Lönnqvist J, et al. The genetic epidemiology of schizophrenia in a Finnish twin cohort: a population-based modeling study. *JAMA Psychiatry*. 1998;55:67–74. https://doi.org/10.1001/archpsyc.55.1.67.

35. Jones P, Cannon M. The new epidemiology of schizophrenia. *Psychiatr Clin N Am*. 1998;21:1–25.

36. Heston LL. Psychiatric disorders in foster home reared children of schizophrenic mothers. *Br J Psychiatry*. 1966;112:819–825. https://doi.org/10.1192/bjp.112.489.819.

37. Kety SS, Wender PH, Jacobsen B, et al. Mental illness in the biological and adoptive relatives of schizophrenic adoptees. Replication of the Copenhagen Study in the rest of Denmark. *Arch Gen Psychiatry*. 1994;51:442–455. https://doi.org/10.1001/archpsyc.1994.03950060006001.

38. Kety SS. Schizophrenic illness in the families of schizophrenic adoptees: findings from the Danish national sample. *Schizophr Bull*. 1988;14:217–222. https://doi.org/10.1093/schbul/14.2.217.

39. Wahlberg KE, Wynne LC, Oja H, et al. Gene-environment interaction in vulnerability to schizophrenia: findings from the Finnish Adoptive Family Study of Schizophrenia. *Am J Psychiatry*. 1997;154:355–362. https://doi.org/10.1176/ajp.154.3.355.

40. Zhuo C, Hou W, Lin C, et al. Potential value of genomic copy number variations in schizophrenia. *Front Mol Neurosci*. 2017;10:204. https://doi.org/10.3389/fnmol.2017.00204.

41. Girirajan S, Campbell CD, Eichler EE. Human copy number variation and complex genetic disease. *Annu Rev Genet*. 2011;45:203–226. https://doi.org/10.1146/annurev-genet-102209-163544.

42. Lowther C, Merico D, Costain G, et al. Impact of IQ on the diagnostic yield of chromosomal microarray in a community sample of adults with schizophrenia. *Genome Med*. 2017;9:105. https://doi.org/10.1186/s13073-017-0488-z.

43. Malaspina D, Goetz RR, Friedman JH, et al. Traumatic brain injury and schizophrenia in members of schizophrenia and bipolar disorder pedigrees. *Am J Psychiatry*. 2001;158:440–446. https://doi.org/10.1176/appi.ajp.158.3.440.

44. Malaspina D, Harlap S, Fennig S, et al. Advancing paternal age and the risk of schizophrenia. *Arch Gen Psychiatry*. 2001;58:361–367.

45. El-Saadi O, Pedersen CB, McNeil TF, et al. Paternal and maternal age as risk factors for psychosis: findings from Denmark. *Sweden and Australia Schizophr Res*. 2004;67:227–236. https://doi.org/10.1016/S0920-9964(03)00100-2.

46. Sipos A, Rasmussen F, Harrison G, et al. Paternal age and schizophrenia: a population based cohort study. *BMJ*. 2004;329:1070. https://doi.org/10.1136/bmj.38243.672396.55.
47. Malaspina D, Corcoran C, Fahim C, et al. Paternal age and sporadic schizophrenia: evidence for de novo mutations. *Am J Med Genet*. 2002;114:299–303. https://doi.org/10.1002/ajmg.1701.
48. Malaspina D, Friedman JH, Kaufmann C, et al. Psychobiological heterogeneity of familial and sporadic schizophrenia. *Biol Psychiatry*. 1998;43:489–496. https://doi.org/10.1016/s0006-3223(97)00527-1.
49. Izumoto Y, Inoue S, Yasuda N. Schizophrenia and the influenza epidemics of 1957 in Japan. *Biol Psychiatry*. 1999;46:119–124. https://doi.org/10.1016/s0006-3223(98)00359-x.
50. O'Callaghan E, Sham P, Takei N, et al. Schizophrenia after prenatal exposure to 1957 A2 influenza epidemic. *Lancet (London, England)*. 1991;337:1248–1250. https://doi.org/10.1016/0140-6736(91)92919-s.
51. Mehta D, Tropf FC, Gratten J, et al. Evidence for genetic overlap between schizophrenia and age at first birth in women. *JAMA Psychiatry*. 2016;73:497–505. https://doi.org/10.1001/jamapsychiatry.2016.0129.
52. Byars SG, Boomsma JJ. Opposite differential risks for autism and schizophrenia based on maternal age, paternal age, and parental age differences. *Evol Med Public Health*. 2016;2016:286–298. https://doi.org/10.1093/emph/eow023.
53. Brown AS, Cohen P, Greenwald S, et al. Nonaffective psychosis after prenatal exposure to rubella. *Am J Psychiatry*. 2000;157:438–443. https://doi.org/10.1176/appi.ajp.157.3.438.
54. Brown AS, Schaefer CA, Wyatt RJ, et al. Maternal exposure to respiratory infections and adult schizophrenia spectrum disorders: a prospective birth cohort study. *Schizophr Bull*. 2000;26:287–295. https://doi.org/10.1093/oxfordjournals.schbul.a033453.
55. David AS, Prince M. Psychosis following head injury: a critical review. *J Neurol Neurosurg Psychiatry*. 2005;76(Suppl 1):i53–i60. https://doi.org/10.1136/jnnp.2004.060475.
56. Suvisaari J, Haukka J, Tanskanen A, et al. Association between prenatal exposure to poliovirus infection and adult schizophrenia. *Am J Psychiatry*. 1999;156:1100–1102. https://doi.org/10.1176/ajp.156.7.1100.
57. Erlenmeyer-Kimling L, Folnegovic Z, Hrabak-Zerjavic V, et al. Schizophrenia and prenatal exposure to the 1957 A2 influenza epidemic in Croatia. *Am J Psychiatry*. 1994;151:1496–1498. https://doi.org/10.1176/ajp.151.10.1496.
58. Kelleher I, Keeley H, Corcoran P, et al. Childhood trauma and psychosis in a prospective cohort study: cause, effect, and directionality. *Am J Psychiatry*. 2013;170:734–741. https://doi.org/10.1176/appi.ajp.2012.12091169.
59. Bembenek A. Seasonality of birth in schizophrenia patients. Literature review. *Psychiatr Pol*. 2005;39:259–270.
60. Brown AS, Cohen P, Harkavy-Friedman J, et al. Prenatal rubella, premorbid abnormalities, and adult schizophrenia. *Biol Psychiatry*. 2001;49:473–486. https://doi.org/10.1016/S0006-3223(01)01068-X.
61. Brown AS, Begg MD, Gravenstein S, et al. Serologic evidence of prenatal influenza in the etiology of schizophrenia. *Arch Gen Psychiatry*. 2004;61:774–780. https://doi.org/10.1001/archpsyc.61.8.774.
62. Fuglewicz AJ, Piotrowski P, Stodolak A. Relationship between toxoplasmosis and schizophrenia: a review. *Adv Clin Exp Med*. 2017;26:1031–1036. https://doi.org/10.17219/acem/61435.
63. Rantakallio P, Jones P, Moring J, et al. Association between central nervous system infections during childhood and adult onset schizophrenia and other psychoses: a 28-year follow-up. *Int J Epidemiol*. 1997;26:837–843. https://doi.org/10.1093/ije/26.4.837.
64. Cannon TD, van Erp TGM, Rosso IM, et al. Fetal hypoxia and structural brain abnormalities in schizophrenic patients, their siblings, and controls. *JAMA Psychiatry*. 2002;59:35–41. https://doi.org/10.1001/archpsyc.59.1.35.
65. Hunter A, Murray R, Asher L, et al. The effects of tobacco smoking, and prenatal tobacco smoke exposure, on risk of schizophrenia: a systematic review and meta-analysis. *Nicotine Tob Res*. 2018. https://doi.org/10.1093/ntr/nty160.
66. Palmer CGS, Mallery E, Turunen JA, et al. Effect of Rhesus D incompatibility on schizophrenia depends on offspring sex. *Schizophr Res*. 2008;104:135–145. https://doi.org/10.1016/j.schres.2008.06.022.
67. Fineberg AM, Ellman LM, Schaefer CA, et al. Fetal exposure to maternal stress and risk for schizophrenia spectrum disorders among offspring: differential influences of fetal sex. *Psychiatry Res*. 2016;236:91–97. https://doi.org/10.1016/j.psychres.2015.12.026.
68. Stein AD, Pierik FH, Verrips GHW, et al. Maternal exposure to the Dutch famine before conception and during pregnancy: quality of life and depressive symptoms in adult offspring. *Epidemiology*. 2009;20:909–915. https://doi.org/10.1097/EDE.0b013e3181b5f227.

69. Xu M-Q, Sun W-S, Liu B-X, et al. Prenatal malnutrition and adult schizophrenia: further evidence from the 1959-1961 Chinese famine. *Schizophr Bull.* 2009;35:568–576. https://doi.org/10.1093/schbul/sbn168.

70. Bender KG, Azeem N, Morrice J. Schizophrenia and birth order in Pakistan. *Schizophr Res.* 2000;44:113–120. https://doi.org/10.1016/S0920-9964(99)00221-2.

71. Kemppainen L, Veijola J, Jokelainen J, et al. Birth order and risk for schizophrenia: a 31-year follow-up of the Northern Finland 1966 Birth Cohort. *Acta Psychiatr Scand.* 2001;104:148–152. https://doi.org/10.1034/j.1600-0447.2001.00258.x.

72. Robillard PY, Hulsey TC, Perianin J, et al. Association of pregnancy-induced hypertension with duration of sexual cohabitation before conception. *Lancet (London, England).* 1994;344:973–975. https://doi.org/10.1016/s0140-6736(94)91638-1.

73. Bebbington P, Jonas S, Kuipers E, et al. Childhood sexual abuse and psychosis: data from a cross-sectional national psychiatric survey in England. *Br J Psychiatry.* 2011;199(1):29–37. https://doi.org/10.1192/bjp.bp.110.083642.

74. Kelleher I, Keeley H, Corcoran P, et al. Childhood trauma and psychosis in a prospective cohort study: cause, effect, and directionality. *Am J Psychiatry.* 2013;170(7):734–741. https://doi.org/10.1176/appi.ajp.2012.12091169.

75. Brown AS, Schaefer CA, Wyatt RJ, et al. Maternal exposure to respiratory infections and adult schizophrenia spectrum disorders: a prospective birth cohort study. *Schizophr Bull.* 2000;26(2):287–295. https://doi.org/10.1093/oxfordjournals.schbul.a033453.

76. Brown AS. The environment and susceptibility to schizophrenia. *Progress in Neurobiology.* 2011;93(1):23–58. https://doi.org/10.1016/j.pneurobio.2010.09.003.

77. Sorensen HJ, Mortensen EL, Reinisch JM, et al. Association between prenatal exposure to analgesics and risk of schizophrenia. *Br J Psychiatry.* 2004;185:366–371. https://doi.org/10.1192/bjp.185.5.366.

78. Larkin W, Read J. Childhood trauma and psychosis: evidence, pathways, and implications. *J Postgrad Med.* 2008;54:287–293.

79. Addington J, Farris M, Stowkowy J, et al. Predictors of transition to psychosis in individuals at clinical high risk. *Curr Psychiatry Rep.* 2019;21:39. https://doi.org/10.1007/s11920-019-1027-y.

80. Egerton A, Howes OD, Houle S, et al. Elevated striatal dopamine function in immigrants and their children: a risk mechanism for psychosis. *Schizophr Bull.* 2017;43:293–301. https://doi.org/10.1093/schbul/sbw181.

81. Messias EL, Chen C-Y, Eaton WW. Epidemiology of schizophrenia: review of findings and myths. *Psychiatr Clin North Am.* 2007;30:323–338. https://doi.org/10.1016/j.psc.2007.04.007.

82. Carney R, Cotter J, Firth J, et al. Cannabis use and symptom severity in individuals at ultra high risk for psychosis: a meta-analysis. *Acta Psychiatr Scand.* 2017;136:5–15. https://doi.org/10.1111/acps.12699.

83. Kraan T, Velthorst E, Koenders L, et al. Cannabis use and transition to psychosis in individuals at ultra-high risk: review and meta-analysis. *Psychol Med.* 2016;46:673–681. https://doi.org/10.1017/S0033291715002329.

84. Green MF. What are the functional consequences of neurocognitive deficits in schizophrenia? *Am J Psychiatry.* 1996;153:321–330. https://doi.org/10.1176/ajp.153.3.321.

85. Abi-Dargham A. Do we still believe in the dopamine hypothesis? New data bring new evidence. *Int J Neuropsychopharmacol.* 2004;7(Suppl 1):S1–S5. https://doi.org/10.1017/S1461145704004110.

86. Schobel SA, Lewandowski NM, Corcoran CM, et al. Differential targeting of the CA1 subfield of the hippocampal formation by schizophrenia and related psychotic disorders. *Arch Gen Psychiatry.* 2009;66:938–946. https://doi.org/10.1001/archgenpsychiatry.2009.115.

87. Li P, Snyder GL, Vanover KE. Dopamine targeting drugs for the treatment of schizophrenia: past, present and future. *Curr Top Med Chem.* 2016;16:3385–3403. https://doi.org/10.2174/1568026616666160608084834.

88. Goff DC, Coyle JT. The emerging role of glutamate in the pathophysiology and treatment of schizophrenia. *Am J Psychiatry.* 2001;158:1367–1377. https://doi.org/10.1176/appi.ajp.158.9.1367.

89. Lodge DJ, Grace AA. Hippocampal dysregulation of dopamine system function and the pathophysiology of schizophrenia. *Trends Pharmacol Sci.* 2011;32:507–513. https://doi.org/10.1016/j.tips.2011.05.001.

90. Santos E, Noggle CA. Synaptic pruning. In: Goldstein S, Naglieri JA, eds. *Encyclopedia of Child Behavior and Development.* Boston, MA: Springer US; 2011:1464–1465.

91. Petanjek Z, Judaš M, Šimić G, et al. Extraordinary neoteny of synaptic spines in the human prefrontal cortex. *Proc Natl Acad Sci USA.* 2011;108:13281-LP–13286. https://doi.org/10.1073/pnas.1105108108.

92. Connor CM, Crawford BC, Akbarian S. White matter neuron alterations in schizophrenia and related disorders. *Int J Dev Neurosci.* 2011;29:325–334. https://doi.org/10.1016/j.ijdevneu.2010.07.236.

93. Glausier JR, Lewis DA. Dendritic spine pathology in schizophrenia. *Neuroscience.* 2013;251:90–107. https://doi.org/10.1016/j.neuroscience.2012.04.044.

94. Osimo EF, Beck K, Reis Marques T, et al. Synaptic loss in schizophrenia: a meta-analysis and systematic review of synaptic protein and mRNA measures. *Mol Psychiatry.* 2019;24:549–561. https://doi.org/10.1038/s41380-018-0041-5.

95. Glantz LA, Lewis DA. Decreased dendritic spine density on prefrontal cortical pyramidal neurons in schizophrenia. *Arch Gen Psychiatry.* 2000;57:65–73.

96. Konopaske GT, Lange N, Coyle JT, et al. Prefrontal cortical dendritic spine pathology in schizophrenia and bipolar disorder. *JAMA Psychiatry.* 2014;71:1323–1331. https://doi.org/10.1001/jamapsychiatry.2014.1582.

97. Sellgren CM, Gracias J, Watmuff B, et al. Increased synapse elimination by microglia in schizophrenia patient-derived models of synaptic pruning. *Nat Neurosci.* 2019;22:374–385. https://doi.org/10.1038/s41593-018-0334-7.

98. Wang X, Christian KM, Song H, et al. Synaptic dysfunction in complex psychiatric disorders: from genetics to mechanisms. *Genome Med.* 2018;10:9. https://doi.org/10.1186/s13073-018-0518-5.

99. Mubarik A, Tohid H. Frontal lobe alterations in schizophrenia: a review. *Trends Psychiatry Psychother.* 2016;38:198–206. https://doi.org/10.1590/2237-6089-2015-0088.

100. Shepherd AM, Quide Y, Laurens KR, et al. Shared intermediate phenotypes for schizophrenia and bipolar disorder: neuroanatomical features of subtypes distinguished by executive dysfunction. *J Psychiatry Neurosci.* 2015;40:58–68.

101. Cardno AG, Marshall EJ, Coid B, et al. Heritability estimates for psychotic disorders: the Maudsley twin psychosis series. *Arch Gen Psychiatry.* 1999;56:162–168. https://doi.org/10.1001/archpsyc.56.2.162.

102. Lyngberg K, Buchy L, Liu L, et al. Patterns of premorbid functioning in individuals at clinical high risk of psychosis. *Schizophr Res.* 2015;169:209–213. https://doi.org/10.1016/j.schres.2015.11.004.

103. Zarogianni E, Storkey AJ, Borgwardt S, et al. Individualized prediction of psychosis in subjects with an at-risk mental state. *Schizophr Res.* 2017. https://doi.org/10.1016/j.schres.2017.08.061.

104. Zarogianni E, Storkey AJ, Johnstone EC, et al. Improved individualized prediction of schizophrenia in subjects at familial high risk, based on neuroanatomical data, schizotypal and neurocognitive features. *Schizophr Res.* 2017;181:6–12. https://doi.org/10.1016/j.schres.2016.08.027.

105. Das T, Borgwardt S, Hauke DJ, et al. Disorganized gyrification network properties during the transition to psychosis. *JAMA Psychiatry.* 2018;75:613–622. https://doi.org/10.1001/jamapsychiatry.2018.0391.

106. Anticevic A, Haut K, Murray JD, et al. Association of thalamic dysconnectivity and conversion to psychosis in youth and young adults at elevated clinical risk. *JAMA Psychiatry.* 2015;72:882–891. https://doi.org/10.1001/jamapsychiatry.2015.0566.

107. Bodatsch M, Brockhaus-Dumke A, Klosterkotter J, et al. Forecasting psychosis by event-related potentials-systematic review and specific meta-analysis. *Biol Psychiatry.* 2015;77:951–958. https://doi.org/10.1016/j.biopsych.2014.09.025.

108. Tang Y, Wang J, Zhang T, et al. P300 as an index of transition to psychosis and of remission: data from a clinical high risk for psychosis study and review of literature. *Schizophr Res.* 2019. https://doi.org/10.1016/j.schres.2019.02.014.

109. Battaglia M, Cavallini MC, Macciardi F, et al. The structure of DSM-III-R schizotypal personality disorder diagnosed by direct interviews. *Schizophr Bull.* 1997;23:83–92. https://doi.org/10.1093/schbul/23.1.83.

110. Maier W, Lichtermann D, Minges J, et al. Personality disorders among the relatives of schizophrenia patients. *Schizophr Bull.* 1994;20:481–493. https://doi.org/10.1093/schbul/20.3.481.

111. Ross RG, Olincy A, Harris JG, et al. Smooth pursuit eye movements in schizophrenia and attentional dysfunction: adults with schizophrenia, ADHD, and a normal comparison group. *Biol Psychiatry.* 2000;48:197–203. https://doi.org/10.1016/s0006-3223(00)00825-8.

112. Klar AA, Ballmaier M, Leopold K, et al. Interaction of hippocampal volume and N-acetylaspartate concentration deficits in schizophrenia: a combined MRI and 1H-MRS study. *Neuroimage.* 2010;53:51–57. https://doi.org/10.1016/j.neuroimage.2010.06.006.

113. Pujol N, Penadés R, Junqué C, et al. Hippocampal abnormalities and age in chronic schizophrenia: morphometric study across the adult lifespan. *Br J Psychiatry.* 2014;205:369–375. https://doi.org/10.1192/bjp.bp.113.140384.

114. Santos JL, Sanchez-Morla EM, Aparicio A, et al. P50 gating in deficit and nondeficit schizophrenia. *Schizophr Res*. 2010;119:183–190. https://doi.org/10.1016/j.schres.2010.01.010.
115. Forbes NF, Carrick LA, McIntosh AM, et al. Working memory in schizophrenia: a meta-analysis. *Psychol Med*. 2009. https://doi.org/10.1017/S0033291708004558.
116. Millard SP, Shofer J, Braff D, et al. Prioritizing schizophrenia endophenotypes for future genetic studies: an example using data from the COGS-1 family study. *Schizophr Res*. 2016;174:1–9. https://doi.org/10.1016/j.schres.2016.04.011.
117. Budnik V, Ruiz-Cañada C, Wendler F. Extracellular vesicles round off communication in the nervous system. *Nat Rev Neurosci*. 2016;17:160–172. https://doi.org/10.1038/nrn.2015.29.
118. Saeedi S, Israel S, Nagy C, et al. The emerging role of exosomes in mental disorders. *Transl Psychiatry*. 2019;9:122. https://doi.org/10.1038/s41398-019-0459-9.
119. Fish B. Biologic antecedents of psychosis in children. *Res Publ Assoc Res Nerv Ment Dis*. 1975;54:49–83.
120. Tripathi A, Kar SK, Shukla R. Cognitive deficits in schizophrenia: understanding the biological correlates and remediation strategies. *Clin Psychopharmacol Neurosci*. 2018;16:7–17. https://doi.org/10.9758/cpn.2018.16.1.7.
121. Walker E, Lewis N, Loewy R, et al. Motor dysfunction and risk for schizophrenia. *Dev Psychopathol*. 1999;11:509–523.
122. Walker EF, Savoie T, Davis D. Neuromotor precursors of schizophrenia. *Schizophr Bull*. 1994;20:441–451. https://doi.org/10.1093/schbul/20.3.441.
123. Pallanti S, Quercioli L, Pazzagli A. Social anxiety and premorbid personality disorders in paranoid schizophrenic patients treated with clozapine. *CNS Spectr*. 2000;5:29–43. https://doi.org/10.1017/S1092852900021635.
124. Erlenmeyer-Kimling L, Cornblatt BA. A summary of attentional findings in the New York high-risk project. *J Psychiatr Res*. 1992;26:405–426. https://doi.org/10.1016/0022-3956(92)90043-N.
125. Parnas J, Schulsinger F, Schulsinger H, Mednick SA, Teasdale TW. Behavioral precursors of schizophrenia spectrum. A prospective study. *Arch Gen Psychiatry*. 1982;39(6):658–664. https://doi.org/10.1001/archpsyc.1982.04290060020005.
126. Bartlett J. Childhood-onset schizophrenia: what do we really know? *Heal Psychol Behav Med*. 2014;2:735–747. https://doi.org/10.1080/21642850.2014.927738.
127. Cicchetti D, Toth SL. Child maltreatment. *Annu Rev Clin Psychol*. 2004;1:409–438. https://doi.org/10.1146/annurev.clinpsy.1.102803.144029.
128. Li X-B, Li Q-Y, Liu J-T, et al. Childhood trauma associates with clinical features of schizophrenia in a sample of Chinese inpatients. *Psychiatry Res*. 2015;228:702–707. https://doi.org/10.1016/j.psychres.2015.06.001.
129. Schenkel LS, Spaulding WD, DiLillo D, et al. Histories of childhood maltreatment in schizophrenia: relationships with premorbid functioning, symptomatology, and cognitive deficits. *Schizophr Res*. 2005;76:273–286. https://doi.org/10.1016/j.schres.2005.03.003.
130. Hall W, Degenhardt L. Cannabis use and the risk of developing a psychotic disorder. *World Psychiatry*. 2008;7:68–71.
131. Pantelis C, Yucel M, Wood SJ, et al. Structural brain imaging evidence for multiple pathological processes at different stages of brain development in schizophrenia. *Schizophr Bull*. 2005;31:672–696. https://doi.org/10.1093/schbul/sbi034.
132. Kasai K, Shenton ME, Salisbury DF, et al. Progressive decrease of left superior temporal gyrus gray matter volume in patients with first-episode schizophrenia. *Am J Psychiatry*. 2003;160:156–164. https://doi.org/10.1176/appi.ajp.160.1.156.

CHAPTER 3

Obsessive-Compulsive Schizophrenia and Obsessive-Compulsive Disorder

Michael Poyurovsky ■ Michael Hwang

Abstract

Schizophrenia and obsessive-compulsive disorder (OCD) are distinct nosologic entities, but they overlap in their demographic and clinical characteristics and in aspects of their neurobiological underpinnings and treatment. Both are chronic disorders associated with periods of exacerbation and remission; both affect men and women equally and have a similar age-at-onset distribution, with an earlier age of onset for men in both conditions. The two disorders share a common neurobiological background and therapeutic approaches. Hence it is not surprising that OCD has been identified in a clinically significant proportion of schizophrenia patients, or that it may play a central role in some cases. This chapter focuses primarily on clinical and psychopathologic aspects of the complex psychiatric disorder of obsessive-compulsive schizophrenia. Included are some tips for diagnostic interviewing patients for comorbid schizophrenia and OCD, a clinical vignette that illustrates diagnostic challenges and treatment response, and pharmacotherapy approaches and challenges.

KEYWORDS

Comorbidity   Insight   Obsessive-compulsive   Schizophrenia

Introduction

In the current psychiatric classifications, schizophrenia and obsessive-compulsive disorder (OCD) are regarded as distinct clinical entities characterized by specific diagnostic criteria, clinical presentations, prognosis, and treatment. Nevertheless, they share some demographic and clinical characteristics as well as underlying pathophysiologic mechanisms. The two disorders have similar prevalence estimates, gender distributions, age at onset, and course of illness. Neuropathologic and neuroimaging studies show a substantial overlap between schizophrenia and OCD in structural and functional brain abnormalities and in the involvement of dopamine, serotonin, and glutamate neurotransmitter systems in the pathophysiology underlying these disorders. Thus, it is not surprising that OCD occurs in a substantially higher proportion of schizophrenia patients than would be expected by chance (Table 3.1).

TABLE 3.1 ▪ Schematic Comparative Characteristics of Schizophrenia and Obsessive-Compulsive Disorder

	Schizophrenia	OCD
Prevalence	~ 1%, narrowly defined 2%–3%, broadly defined	2%–3%
Gender ratio (M/F)	1/1	1/1
Age of onset	2nd–3rd decade Men earlier than women	2nd–3rd decade Men earlier than women
Course	Chronic with remissions	Chronic, wax and wane
Involved brain regions	Cortex: DLPC, temporal, ACC; thalamus, hippocampus, striatum	Cortex: OFC, ACC; thalamus, striatum
Neurotransmitter systems	Dopamine/serotonin/glutamate	Serotonin/dopamine/glutamate
Treatment	Antipsychotic agents (add-on serotonin reuptake inhibitors)	Serotonin reuptake inhibitors (add-on antipsychotic agents)

ACC, Anterior cingulate cortex; DLPC, dorsolateral prefrontal cortex; OCD, obsessive-compulsive disorder; OFC, orbitofrontal cortex.

This chapter focuses on the clinical characterization of the complex psychopathologic interface between schizophrenia and OCD, sometimes considered "obsessive-compulsive schizophrenia" (OC-SCZ). This chapter is a guide to improving early recognition, differential diagnosis, and treatment of this complex psychiatric disorder.

Schizophrenia

According to DSM-5 criteria, the diagnosis of schizophrenia is based on a constellation of positive, negative, and disorganized symptoms, illness duration (at least 6 months, including at least 1 month of active phase), and functional impairment, after exclusion of affective disorders, and psychotic disorders associated with substance abuse or general medical conditions.[1] Psychopathologic symptoms of schizophrenia are differentially expressed among different patients and different phases of illness.[2] Although various delusions might occur within the positive symptom dimension, a majority of patients exhibit a restricted set of typical delusional themes (e.g., reference, persecution, grandeur, somatic, guilt, jealousy). Hallucinations can occur in any of the sensory modalities, though auditory hallucinations, imperative voices commenting or conversing, are far more common. Formal thought disorders refer to disorganization of the logical and goal-directed thought process, and range in severity from mild circumstantiality, tangentiality, derailment, and neologisms to severe incoherence.[3]

Negative symptoms are intrinsic to schizophrenia and include restricted and blunted affect, anhedonia, avolition, apathy, and alogia.[4] Negative symptoms may be detected at every stage of illness, including prodromal, acute, and chronic, and are strongly associated with functional impairment. Motor symptoms of schizophrenia include slowness, complex stereotypic movements, mannerisms, and catatonic symptoms. Affective symptoms are common and may be part of the prodromal phase, follow an acute episode, or occur during remission from schizophrenia. Depressive symptoms substantially contribute to the disease burden and are strongly associated with suicidality in schizophrenia patients (Table 3.2).

TABLE 3.2 ■ **Diagnostic Criteria: Schizophrenia**

DSM5: 295.90 (ICD10: F20.9)

A. Two (or more) of the following, each present for a significant portion of time during a 1-month period (or less if successfully treated). At least one of these must be (1), (2), or (3):
   1. Delusions.
   2. Hallucinations.
   3. Disorganized speech (e.g., frequent derailment or incoherence).
   4. Grossly disorganized or catatonic behavior.
   5. Negative symptoms (i.e., diminished emotional expression or avolition).

B. For a significant portion of the time since the onset of the disturbance, level of functioning in one or more major areas, such as work, interpersonal relations, or self-care, is markedly below the level achieved prior to the onset (or when the onset is in childhood or adolescence, there is failure to achieve expected level of interpersonal, academic, or occupational functioning).

C. Continuous signs of the disturbance persist for at least 6 months. This 6-month period must include at least 1 month of symptoms (or less if successfully treated) that meet Criterion A (i.e., active-phase symptoms) and may include periods of prodromal or residual symptoms. During these prodromal or residual periods, the signs of the disturbance may be manifested by only negative symptoms or by two or more symptoms listed in Criterion A present in an attenuated form (e.g., odd beliefs, unusual perceptual experiences).

D. Schizoaffective disorder and depressive or bipolar disorder with psychotic features have been ruled out because either (1) no major depressive or manic episodes have occurred concurrently with the active-phase symptoms, or (2) if mood episodes have occurred during active-phase symptoms, they have been present for a minority of the total duration of the active and residual periods of the illness.

E. The disturbance is not attributable to the physiologic effects of a substance (e.g., a drug of abuse, a medication) or another medical condition.

F. If there is a history of autism spectrum disorder or a communication disorder of childhood onset, the additional diagnosis of schizophrenia is made only if prominent delusions or hallucinations, in addition to the other required symptoms of schizophrenia, are also present for at least 1 month (or less if successfully treated).

Schizophrenia (page 87—code 295.90, F20.9).
American Psychiatric Association. Schizophrenia spectrum and other psychotic disorders. In *Diagnostic and Statistical Manual of Mental Disorders*. 5th ed. 2013. https://doi.org/10.1176/appi.books.9780890425596.dsm02.

Obsessive-Compulsive Disorder

According to DSM-5 criteria, and similar to schizophrenia, OCD is associated with disturbances of thoughts, affect, and motor function. According to DSM-5 criteria, a diagnosis of OCD requires either obsessions or compulsions that are time-consuming, cause distress, and substantially interfere with normal functioning.[1] Typical obsessions and compulsions are repetitive and intrusive in nature, perceived as unwanted and excessive, and are not simply excessive worries about real-life issues.

Notably, the thoughts are recognized as products of patients' own minds, in contrast to the phenomenon of mind reading in schizophrenia. In addition, the obsessive-compulsive (OC) symptoms are not attributable to the physiologic effects of a substance (e.g., a drug of abuse, a medication) or another medical condition (e.g., epilepsy, head trauma), and the disturbance is not better explained by the symptoms of another mental disorder (e.g., eating disorder, anxiety disorder).[1] The content of obsessions differs substantially from patient to patient. However, similar to delusions (with their restricted set of distinctive themes), there are several typical themes of obsessions, namely contamination, symmetry, and forbidden thoughts (aggressive, sexual, religious). Specific obsessions are associated with corresponding compulsions and form psychopathologic dimensions that are relatively stable over time (Table 3.3).[5]

TABLE 3.3 ■ **Diagnostic Criteria: Obsessive-Compulsive Disorder**

DSM-5 300.3 (ICD10 F42.2 F42)

A. Presence of obsessions, compulsions, or both:
- Obsessions are defined by (1) and (2):
  1. Recurrent and persistent thoughts, urges, or images that are experienced, at some time during the disturbance, as intrusive and unwanted, and that in most individuals cause marked anxiety or distress.
  2. The individual attempts to ignore or suppress such thoughts, urges, or images, or to neutralize them with some other thought or action (i.e., by performing a compulsion).
- Compulsions are defined by (1) and (2):
  1. Repetitive behaviors (e.g., handwashing, ordering, checking) or mental acts (e.g., praying, counting, repeating words silently) that the individual feels driven to perform in response to an obsession or according to rules that must be applied rigidly.
  2. The behaviors or mental acts are aimed at preventing or reducing anxiety or distress, or preventing some dreaded event or situation; however, these behaviors or mental acts are not connected in a realistic way with what they are designed to neutralize or prevent, or are clearly excessive.
- **Note:** Young children may not be able to articulate the aims of these behaviors or mental acts.

B. The obsessions or compulsions are time-consuming (e.g., take more than 1 hour/day) or cause clinically significant distress or impairment in social, occupational, or other important areas of functioning.

C. The obsessive-compulsive symptoms are not attributable to the physiologic effects of a substance (e.g., a drug of abuse, a medication) or another medical condition.

D. The disturbance is not better explained by the symptoms of another mental disorder (e.g., excessive worries, as in generalized anxiety disorder; preoccupation with appearance, as in body dysmorphic disorder; difficulty discarding or parting with possessions, as in hoarding disorder; hair pulling, as in trichotillomania [hair-pulling disorder]; skin picking, as in excoriation [skin-picking] disorder; stereotypies, as in stereotypic movement disorder; ritualized eating behavior, as in eating disorders; preoccupation with substances or gambling, as in substance-related and addictive disorders; preoccupation with having an illness, as in illness anxiety disorder; sexual urges or fantasies, as in paraphilic disorders; impulses, as in disruptive, impulse-control, and conduct disorders; guilty ruminations, as in major depressive disorder; thought insertion or delusional preoccupations, as in schizophrenia spectrum and other psychotic disorders; or repetitive patterns of behavior, as in autism spectrum disorder).

Specify if:
With good or fair insight: The individual recognizes that obsessive-compulsive disorder beliefs are definitely or probably not true or that they may or may not be true.
With poor insight: The individual thinks obsessive-compulsive disorder beliefs are probably true.
With absent insight/delusional beliefs: The individual is completely convinced that obsessive-compulsive disorder beliefs are true.

Obsessive-Compulsive Disorder (page 235—code 300.3, F42).
American Psychiatric Association. Obsessive-compulsive and related disorders. In *Diagnostic and Statistical Manual of Mental Disorders*. 5th ed. 2013. https://doi.org/10.1176/appi.books.9780890425596.dsm06.

NEAR-PSYCHOTIC SYMPTOMS IN OBSESSIVE-COMPULSIVE DISORDER

Despite clear-cut differences in psychopathology between schizophrenia and OCD, there is a substantial overlap, a "gray zone," between the two disorders. Thus, unusual and "bizarre" obsessive themes exhibited by a subgroup of otherwise typical OCD patients might complicate the distinction between the obsessions and delusions. The difference between OCD-related pathologic slowness and the restrictive motor output associated with negative symptoms of schizophrenia or with catatonic motor disturbances is not straightforward. The differential diagnosis between OCD-related indecisiveness and pathologic doubt and schizophrenic ambivalence is also challenging. Patient insight into the senseless nature of OC symptoms is one of the hallmarks of the disorder. According to the DSM-5, at some point in the course of the illness, the patients must recognize that their obsessive beliefs are "definitely or probably not true." Indeed, in typical OCD cases, patients readily acknowledge that their OC symptoms are illogical and pathologic.

On the other hand, a significant majority of schizophrenia patients either do not believe that they are ill, or even if they do acknowledge symptoms, they misattribute them to other causes.[6] Nevertheless, a significant subset of OCD patients can sometimes present without insight, or with conviction that their obsessions are true, thus complicating the differential diagnosis of obsessions from delusions.

Overall, from the psychopathologic perspective, schizophrenia and OCD are distinct, despite their partially overlapping characteristics. Some symptoms, such as delusions and obsessions, pathologic doubt and ambivalence, rituals and motor stereotypy, may represent a continuum of OCD impairments, while others, such as negative and disorganized symptoms, are more schizophrenia-specific (Fig 3.1).

OBSESSIVE-COMPULSIVE DISORDER AS A RISK FACTOR FOR SCHIZOPHRENIA

Ample evidence of a close interrelationship between the two disorders comes from epidemiologic studies that convincingly indicate that a diagnosis of OCD confers a risk for later development of schizophrenia.[7-9] In a study based on Danish registries, prior diagnosis of OCD was associated with an

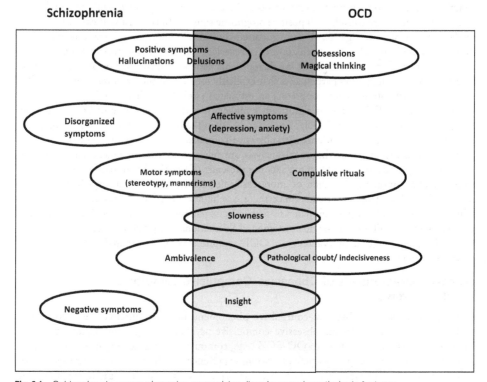

Fig. 3.1   Schizophrenia versus obsessive-compulsive disorder: psychopathologic features.

increased risk of developing schizophrenia (incidence rate ratio [IRR] = 6.90; 95% confidence interval [CI], 6.25–7.60) and schizophrenia spectrum disorders (IRR = 5.77; 95% CI, 5.33–6.22) later in life.[7] Similarly, children of parents with OCD had an increased risk of schizophrenia (IRR = 4.31; 95% CI, 2.72–6.43) and schizophrenia spectrum disorders (IRR = 3.10; 95% CI, 2.17–4.27). A Swedish registry-based longitudinal cohort and multigenerational family study found that patients with OCD had a substantially higher risk of having a comorbid diagnosis of schizophrenia and schizoaffective disorder compared with individuals without OCD.[8] Individuals first diagnosed with OCD had a three fold higher risk of receiving a later diagnosis of schizophrenia compared with individuals without OCD.

From the perspective of psychotic diagnoses, patients first diagnosed with schizophrenia and schizoaffective disorder had a seven- and five-times higher risk of receiving a later diagnosis of OCD, respectively, in comparison with individuals without schizophrenia. A recent large-scale Australian epidemiologic study supports a link between the two disorders by showing a considerably higher risk of schizophrenia in the OCD group compared to matched non-OCD controls (hazard ratio: 30.29, 95%, CI, 17.91–51.21).[9] Notably, male gender, age of OCD onset before 20 years, and antipsychotic prescriptions were associated with schizophrenia. Overall, these well-designed large-scale epidemiologic investigations convincingly demonstrated that it is essential for psychiatrists to be aware that OCD may herald further development of schizophrenia as a pathophysiologically related comorbid disorder, or even as a unique entity, namely OC-SCZ.

OBSESSIVE-COMPULSIVE DISORDER/SYMPTOMS IN SCHIZOPHRENIA

Prevalence

Initially, OC symptoms were thought to occur in a minority of patients with schizophrenia (1.1%–3.5%), and were considered a positive prognostic sign.[10,11] In contrast to these early studies, modern large-scale investigations using structured clinical interviews, and operationally defined diagnostic criteria for OCD and schizophrenia, revealed that obsessive-compulsive phenomena are prevalent and clinically significant in schizophrenia patients. Thus, based on an analysis of 34 studies with more than 3000 participants that explicitly focused on the assessment of OCD/OC symptoms in patients with schizophrenia, an estimated pooled prevalence of OCD in schizophrenia was 12.1%.[12] This rate is significantly higher than the lifetime rate of OCD found in the general population (1.3%–2.3%).[13] Importantly, when the diagnostic threshold is relaxed, the proportion of schizophrenia patients with obsessive-compulsive symptoms rises to 25%.[12]

Several conclusions from this meta-analysis are relevant to clinical practice. For patients with acute psychosis, it is useful to reassess the presence of OCD after resolution of psychosis, since OCD symptoms might then be more easily detectable, which could explain the higher rates of OCD found in outpatients. Since there is a higher prevalence of OCD after repeated schizophrenia episodes, when compared to first-episode patients, it may be that OCD rates may increase over time. This could be due to temporal fluctuations, antipsychotic treatment, or other factors. Ongoing longitudinal evaluation of OCD symptoms is thus warranted during the course of schizophrenic illness.

Clinical Characteristics of Obsessive-Compulsive Symptoms in Schizophrenia

Notably, complexity of obsessive-compulsive phenomena in schizophrenia goes beyond the typical OC symptoms. Unique obsessive-compulsive psychopathologic complexes have been found exclusively in patients with OC-SCZ (e.g., compulsive handwashing due to command auditory hallucinations; ego-dystonic obsessions experienced as thought insertions or auditory hallucinations).[14–16] In view of the fact that these complex psychopathologic features are not captured by currently used diagnostic instruments (e.g., Yale Brown Obsessive Compulsive

Scale, YBOCS),[17] it is plausible that the overall prevalence of obsessive-compulsive features in schizophrenia is underestimated at present.

Similar to their OCD counterparts, a majority of patients with OC-SCZ have both obsessions and compulsions, while a few patients having mono-symptomatic OCD.[18,19] The most frequently observed obsessions are aggressive, contamination, somatic, and symmetry, and the most frequently observed compulsions are checking, cleaning/washing, ordering/arranging, and counting.[20,21] Factor analytic studies exploring an underlying structure of OC symptoms in schizophrenia point toward the existence of five psychopathologic dimensions that resemble those found in "pure" OCD.[20] The first factor *(forbidden thoughts)* includes aggressive, sexual, and religious obsessions and counting compulsions; the second factor *(symmetry)* includes symmetry obsessions and ordering compulsions; the third factor *(cleaning)* includes contamination obsessions and cleaning compulsions; the fourth factor *(somatic)* includes somatic obsessions and repeating compulsions; the fifth factor *(hoarding)* includes hoarding obsessions and checking and repeating compulsions. Temporal stability of these factors in patients with OC-SCZ has not yet been determined.

The mean severity of OC symptoms in OC-SCZ patients is substantial and ranges from moderate to severe (total Y-BOCS = 16 to 40).[22] OC symptom severity seems to progress during the course of schizophrenia, and there is indeed a positive correlation between duration of schizophrenia and severity of OC symptoms.[23] Notably, the relationship between OC symptoms and specific schizophrenia subtypes is less clear. Although there is some indication of more frequent OC symptoms in patients with paranoid, schizo-affective, or undifferentiated subtypes of schizophrenia, a majority of studies failed to reveal predominance association with any specific subtype of schizophrenia.[24,25]

Likewise, reports concerning OC symptom effects on schizophrenia symptom severity are inconsistent. Some studies, primarily those investigating recent-onset schizophrenia, show lower severity of delusions, formal thought disorder, and anergia.[18,26-28] At the same time, other studies have shown higher schizophrenia symptom severity in patients with chronic OC-SCZ.[19,29-31] Most reports, however, do not reveal differences in schizophrenia symptom severity as a function of comorbid OCD.[21,25,32] Differences in study design, sample sizes, and assessment instruments and the inclusion of diverse patient populations may account, at least in part, for these discrepancies.

A meta-analysis that aimed to clarify the effect of OCD/OC symptoms on the severity of schizophrenia symptoms found that the presence of OC symptoms was associated with higher global, positive, and negative symptoms.[33] Overall, the finding of a greater severity of psychosis in OC-SCZ is in line with poorer social and vocational functioning and poorer prognosis in this subset of schizophrenia patients.[34]

INSIGHT IN PATIENTS WITH OBSESSIVE-COMPULSIVE SCHIZOPHRENIA

Insight has consistently been considered one of the key distinguishing features between obsessive-compulsive and psychotic phenomena. Nevertheless, studies demonstrate that patients with OCD may exhibit varying degrees of insight into the validity of their beliefs ranging from lack of insight to full insight.[35] Poor insight was found in a substantial proportion (up to 40%) of OCD patients.[36] DSM-5 acknowledges this phenomenon and adds the following specifier:[1] *with good or fair insight:* the individual recognizes that OCD beliefs are definitely or probably not true or that they may or may not be true; *with poor insight:* the individual thinks OCD beliefs are probably true; *with absent insight/delusional beliefs:* the individual is completely convinced that OCD beliefs are true.

Extensive research into the category of insight, using standardized instruments for the evaluation of awareness of schizophrenia (Scale to Assess Unawareness of Mental Disorder)[37] and insight into OCD (The Brown Assessment of Beliefs Scale),[38] shows that a majority of patients with OC-SCZ have good or fair insight into OC symptoms, which makes them distinguishable from psychotic symptoms.[39] In some cases, however, OC symptoms are characterized not by insight, but rather by full conviction and belief. Moreover, during psychotic exacerbations, obsessions might transform into delusional content and form complex psychopathologic phenomena that incorporate both obsessive-compulsive and other psychotic elements.

These patients pose a particular diagnostic challenge. From clinical experience, poor insight obsessions can be differentiated from delusions based on the typical OCD content (e.g., contamination), accompanying compulsions (e.g., checking, ordering), intact perception, and lack of delusional affect. Importantly, high awareness of OC symptoms apparently does not translate into meaningful awareness of psychotic schizophrenia symptoms. In fact, multiple self-awareness indices found no difference between schizophrenia groups with and without OCD, implying that OC symptoms do not significantly modify patients' awareness of psychosis.[39] Considering that poor awareness of schizophrenia is often associated with poor treatment compliance and poorer outcome, improvement of general illness awareness is critical for improving the prognosis of schizophrenia patients with or without OCD.

AGES OF ONSET FOR SCHIZOPHRENIA AND OBSESSIVE-COMPULSIVE DISORDER

Schizophrenia onset age ranges from mid-adolescence to late adulthood, and peaks in early adulthood.[40] OCD age at onset appears to be earlier, with roughly half of all cases beginning in childhood and adolescence.[13] The two disorders each have a remarkably similar earlier age at onset in men than in women.[13,41] Extensive research on age at onset in schizophrenia and OCD clearly demonstrates its clinical and prognostic significance. Patients with earlier age at onset of schizophrenia are more likely to be male, have poor pre-morbid adjustment, lower educational achievement, more evidence of structural brain abnormalities, and greater cognitive impairments and treatment resistance.[42,43] Correspondingly, early-onset OCD has been associated with male predominance, tic disorders, greater symptom severity, and treatment resistance.[44,45] The finding that patients with early onset are more likely to have relatives with the same illness suggests that early age at onset may be related to greater genetic vulnerability.

Comparative evaluation of age at onset of first schizophrenia and OC symptoms in patients with OC-SCZ found that the mean age of OCD onset was earlier than the mean age of schizophrenia onset (mean difference 1.04 years; 95% CI: 0.67–2.15).[46] One study employed a systematic assessment of age at onset of schizophrenic and OC symptoms among 133 patients (97 men, 36 women; mean age 31.1 ± 8.7 years, mean number of hospitalizations 2.9 ± 2.6) who were consecutively hospitalized at Tirat Carmel Mental Health Center (Israel) and who met DSM-IV criteria for both schizophrenic or schizoaffective disorder and OCD.[47] Briefly, age at onset of the first OC symptoms preceded age of onset of first psychotic symptoms (19.1 ± 7.7 years vs. 20.4 ± 5.9 years; $P < .05$). When gender was considered, there was a significantly earlier age of onset of OC symptoms than schizophrenic symptoms in men (18.3 ± 6.5 vs. 19.8 ± 4.8 years, $P < .05$), but not in women (21.2 ± 9.2 vs. 22.1 ± 7.9 years, $P = .55$).

A secondary analysis revealed that in first-episode predominantly drug-naïve schizophrenia patients ($n = 55$) OC symptoms emerged approximately 3 years earlier than psychotic symptoms (18.2 ± 6.2 vs. 21.6 ± 6.2; $P < .05$). Notably, the average age at onset of first psychotic symptoms was significantly earlier in OC-SCZ patients than in their non-OCD schizophrenia counterparts (20.4 ± 5.9 vs. 23.4 ± 6.7 years; $P < .001$). Overall, the earlier age at onset of OC symptoms than schizophrenia symptoms in OC-SCZ patients suggests that they are independent of psychosis and are not subsequent to schizophrenia-related factors (e.g., antipsychotic treatment). If replicated in larger independent samples of OC-SCZ patients, these findings may indicate an accentuated neuro-developmental origin of OC-SCZ disorder, with earlier onset in men.

COURSE OF ILLNESS

OC symptoms may present across the life span in adolescent, adult, and elderly patients with schizophrenia. The course of OC-SCZ is chronic, and the possibility of full remission is relatively low. Symptom severity fluctuates over time, and there are several patterns of onset and progression of the illness. Studies have shown that in a majority of patients with OC-SCZ, OC symptoms precede initial psychotic symptoms in about 40% of patients, may succeed psychosis in 40%, and occur concurrently with psychotic symptoms in around 20%.[48] In a 5-year follow-up of 172 patients admitted with first-episode schizophrenia, 49% had no OC symptoms anytime during the course, 15% had OC symptoms only during the first assessment, 13% had persistent OC symptoms, 7% developed OC symptoms subsequently, and 16% had intermittent OC symptoms, suggesting that the course of OC symptoms is variable.[21]

Based on clinical experience, Hwang et al.[49] described some potential OC symptom trajectories in schizophrenia. OC symptoms may occur during the prodromal phase, preceding the acute phase of schizophrenia, and may resolve or attenuate after the onset of psychosis. Alternatively, OCD that predates the onset of schizophrenia may persist or worsen regardless of schizophrenic illness progression, as an independent but coexisting disorder. Patients in this category may have initially met criteria for OCD, and subsequently developed psychosis that meets criteria for schizophrenia. Finally, OC symptoms that may develop as part of an acute psychosis will typically resolve with overall improvement in psychosis. The diminished OC symptoms may then present as obsessive rumination or obsessive doubt.

THREE OBSESSIVE-COMPULSIVE DISORDER ONSET PATTERNS IN RELATIONSHIP TO SCHIZOPHRENIA

Several patterns of onset sequence of obsessive-compulsive and schizophrenia symptoms point toward the existence of more than one underlying mechanism of their temporal interrelationship. OC symptoms may co-occur with attenuated psychotic symptoms during a prodromal phase of schizophrenia. These subthreshold OCD symptoms can be considered early symptoms of schizophrenia. Alternatively, OC symptoms may precede schizophrenia in the form of full-scale OCD. From the clinical perspective it is important to note that at least some of these patients will be treated with selective serotonin reuptake inhibitors (SSRIs) and might be susceptible to the development of psychosis. Personal and/or family history of schizophrenia-spectrum disorders in patients with primary diagnosis of OCD should alert psychiatrists to increased risk for psychosis.

When OC symptoms follow the occurrence of schizophrenia, they can be associated with the pathophysiologic and psychological changes of schizophrenia. During the continuing course of schizophrenia, psychotic experiences may become a "focus of obsessive preoccupation," giving rise to the appearance of complex psychopathologic phenomena psychotic in content and obsessive in form.[50,51] These cases, though rare, further support the presence of a psychopathologic continuum between obsessive-compulsive and psychotic phenomena.

Finally, OC symptoms in schizophrenia may be a consequence of antipsychotic treatment, given that there are many reports that atypical antipsychotic agents can induce de novo, or exacerbate preexisting OC symptoms in schizophrenia patients.[52]

DEPRESSIVE SYMPTOMS AND SUICIDALITY IN OBSESSIVE-COMPULSIVE SCHIZOPHRENIA

Several studies note the impact of OC symptoms on the depressive dimension among schizophrenia patients. Thus, Szmulewicz et al.[53] showed a positive correlation between suicidality and intensity of OC symptoms (YBOCS, $r = 0.513$, $P = .01$), and with both YBOCS obsession ($r = 0.444$, $P = .01$) and compulsion subscales ($r = 0.433$, $P = .01$) in a study of 65 schizophrenia patients. Moreover, the total YBOCS was also significantly correlated with depressive symptoms ($r = 0.389$, $P = .01$) and with YBOCS score higher than 8, indicating that clinically significant OCD severity of OCD is an independent predictor of suicide attempts. The impact of OCD on suicidality has been confirmed in a study of 246 patients after first-episode psychosis, where presence of OCD ($N = 26$, 10.6%) was associated with more suicidal plans and attempts in the month before hospitalization.[54] In addition, a 5-year longitudinal follow-up of 176 patients with a first-episode psychosis[21] showed that patients with OCD displayed more severe depressive symptoms at admission and during the follow-up.

Overall, OCD/OC symptoms appeared to be associated with depressive symptoms and suicidality among patients with schizophrenia. Even so, none of these studies evaluated depressive symptoms with the Calgary Depression Scale (a questionnaire validated for assessing depressive symptoms while differentiating them from schizophrenia negative symptoms).[55] Clinicians' awareness and repeated clinical assessments with particular focus on depressive dimensions and suicidality are warranted to ensure early recognition and adequate management of these symptoms in OC-SCZ patients.

NEUROPSYCHOLOGICAL PROFILES IN OBSESSIVE-COMPULSIVE SCHIZOPHRENIA

Neuropsychological studies suggest that patients with OC symptoms have diminished executive functioning, cognitive deficits, and increased negative symptoms, as compared to patients with non-OC schizophrenia.[24,56] Hwang et al.[24] showed that patients with OC symptoms completed fewer categories on the Wisconsin Card Sorting Test ($P < .05$) with a greater perseverative error ($P < .01$), as compared to the non-OC symptoms patients. In addition, OC-SCZ had higher negative symptom ratings on psychopathologic assessment with the Positive and Negative Symptoms Scale ($P < .05$) compared to non-OC symptoms patients. Michalopoulou et al.[56] showed that patients with OC schizophrenia had significantly lower processing speed measured by the reading condition of the Stroop test compared to non-OC schizophrenic patients. Overall, this neurocognitive profile suggests greater impairment of the frontal lobe structure and function.

Additional Comorbidities in Obsessive-Compulsive Schizophrenia

A substantial proportion of patients with both schizophrenia and OCD exhibit additional psychiatric disorders during the life span. Panic anxiety (Chapter 4), social anxiety (Chapter 5), major depressive disorders (Chapters 6 and 7), and substance use (see Chapter 8) are frequently diagnosed comorbidities in both schizophrenia[51] and in OCD.[57,58] In addition, OCD has also been strongly associated with such OCD-related DSM-5 disorders as body dysmorphic disorder, hypochondriasis, tic disorders, and eating disorders.[1] Such OCD-comorbid psychiatric conditions as body dysmorphic disorder and tic disorders may share OCD etiologic pathways, while others (e.g., major depression) may represent secondary syndromes.[57,59] Indeed, considerable overlap has been found in the clinical presentation, familial inheritance, basal ganglia dysfunction, and pharmacotherapy between body dysmorphic disorder, tic disorders, and OCD.[60]

If OC symptoms represent a distinct dimension of psychopathology in schizophrenia, there might be a preferential aggregation of OCD-related disorders in patients with OC-SCZ compared to non-OCD schizophrenia. Indeed, comparing two relatively large schizophrenia patient groups with and without OCD (100 patients per group), over half of the patients had at least one additional psychiatric disorder, supporting the high comorbidity of schizophrenia.[61] Major depression was most frequent, followed by anxiety disorders.

Comparing the two groups, there was a robust differentiation with respect to combined OCD-related disorders evaluated in the study. This difference was primarily due to a substantially higher rate of tic disorders and body dysmorphic disorder in the OC-SCZ group, as compared to the non-OCD schizophrenia group. There was also a higher rate of comorbid eating disorders and hypochondriasis in the OC-SCZ group, however this difference became nonsignificant after adjustment for illness age at onset. Overall, combining OCD-related disorders yielded a robust between-group difference in a number of patients with at least one OCD-spectrum disorder (OC-SCZ 30/100 vs. schizophrenia 8/100; OR = 4.35; 95% CI = 2.13 to 11.41; P = .001).

Moreover, patients with two comorbid OCD-spectrum disorders were found only in the OC-SCZ group (8/100 vs. 0/100, χ^2 = 8.33, P = .0039). These findings strongly suggest that there is a specific elevation in the rate of OCD-related disorders in OC-SCZ patients, rather than generally elevated psychopathology. From a clinical perspective, observation of either OCD or OCD-related symptoms supports careful evaluation for all OCD group syndromes.

Obsessive-Compulsive Symptoms in Prodromal Schizophrenia

Current criteria for individuals at ultra-high risk (UHR) of psychosis include one or more of: attenuated psychotic symptoms, brief limited intermittent psychotic symptoms (less than a week, with spontaneous resolution), or trait and state factors (e.g., presence of schizotypal personality traits).[62] However, since most clinical investigations show substantial clinical heterogeneity, many researchers focus on other psychopathologic dimensions that might predict transition to psychotic disorders.[63]

OCD/OC symptoms has been one area of interest. Several studies estimated their prevalence at 8.4% to 20% in UHR populations.[64–67] To date, though, no studies offer significant findings for OCD-related transition risk in UHR individuals. Thus, in a retrospective cohort of 64 UHR subjects, there was a lower risk of psychotic transition rate among the 20% of subjects with OCD (transition rate 0% in the OCD group vs. 22% in the non-OCD group, P > .05).[65] Fontenelle et al.[66] followed up 37 UHR subjects for 7 years and did not report differences in transition to psychosis based on the presence of OCD at baseline. Notably, incident OC symptoms were associated with greater risk of transition to delusional disorder, psychotic disorders not otherwise specified, depression, or bipolar disorder with psychotic features, but not with schizophrenia.

Overall, since OCD/OC symptoms are prevalent in UHR individuals at a rate comparable to that in first-episode and chronic schizophrenia patients, it appears that OCD persists over the full course of schizophrenia.[52,68] Moreover, OC symptoms in the prodromal phase of schizophrenia have been associated with higher severity of positive symptoms, distress, depression, and suicidality.[34] The association of obsessive-compulsive and negative symptoms of schizophrenia is particularly challenging in terms of differential diagnosis, treatment, and prognosis. In a vast majority of schizophrenia patients, OC symptoms continue beyond the prodromal phase of schizophrenia.

Interview and Assessment Guidelines for Obsessive-Compulsive Disorder Screening in Schizophrenia

Formal guidelines do not yet exist for assessment, identification, and management of obsessive-compulsive phenomena in high-risk individuals, or in prodromal or established schizophrenia patients. Based on clinical experience, the following recommendations can be considered:

1. It is essential to screen individuals who are at high risk or in a prodromal stage of psychosis for OCD/OC symptoms owing to their high prevalence and clinical significance. Conversely, inquiry about attenuated psychotic experiences in patients who present with "full-blown" OCD is prudent, especially in individuals who have a family history of either schizophrenia-spectrum disorders or OCD related disorders.

2. Organic causes for both psychotic and OC symptoms should be ruled out. Metabolic, endocrine, or neurologic factors (e.g., Sydenham's chorea, Huntington's disease) can account for both psychotic or OC symptoms and their co-occurrence.[69]

3. Close follow-up is crucial for obsessive-compulsive and attenuated psychotic components that present during a prodromal phase. The validity of the original diagnosis of prodromal syndrome is provisional, and determined over time. There can be progression to psychosis, to another disorder (e.g., affective), to continuing prodrome, or to remission.

4. Assessment of OCD/OC symptoms after schizophrenia onset can be difficult. Patients may be focused on hallucinations and paranoid delusions, and may have impaired cognition or paranoid fears that frustrate even a very careful interview technique. Even so, many patients can describe OC symptoms in response to specific and carefully phrased questions.

5. Some patients may have psychotic-like symptoms that suggest an OCD core. Awareness of these phenomenon, distress, and voluntary reporting suggest an OCD rather than a perceptual core. For example:
   - Difficulty differentiating between repetitive thoughts and voices
   - Repetitive handwashing, checking locked doors, compulsive rituals

6. Other patients may have OCD symptoms so well incorporated into psychotic phenomenology that the degree of OCD contribution is at first inapparent. For example:
   - Eccentric dress (i.e., all white clothing) to ward off feared persecutors
   - Unusual diet (i.e., no tap water) for fear of poison
   - Ritualized behaviors (i.e., eccentric repetitive movements) directed by voices

Comorbid and premorbid OCD/OC symptom histories may be easier to assess after psychosis is diminished by medication. Full lifetime OC symptom history is essential for understanding the illness as a whole.

Treatment of Obsessive-Compulsive Schizophrenia

Patients with OC-SCZ represent a difficult-to-treat subgroup that requires a distinct therapeutic approach. Addition of an adjunctive SSRI can sometimes effect significant benefit. Escitalopram and sertraline may have more benign pharmacokinetic profiles than other SSRIs. SSRI doses are generally higher than for non-psychotic depression, but perhaps not as high as for non-psychotic OCD.

Even so, there are many treatment approaches and challenges to consider with these patients. When is monotherapy with an antipsychotic agent appropriate, and when is it more effective to add anti-obsessive agents (SSRIs or clomipramine)? At what point should anti-obsessive agents be initiated? What are the short- and long-term risks and benefits of antipsychotic-SSRI combinations? Which patients are susceptible to antipsychotic-induced OC symptoms? How should antipsychotic-induced OC symptoms be treated? What is the role of nonpharmacologic (e.g., cognitive-behavioral therapy [CBT]) intervention in the management of patients with OC-SCZ?

MONOTHERAPY WITH ATYPICAL ANTIPSYCHOTICS FOR OBSESSIVE-COMPULSIVE SCHIZOPHRENIA

Typical antipsychotic agents seem to be of limited therapeutic value for patients with OC-SCZ presumably due to their limited serotonergic properties.[70] A majority of reports to date indicate that atypical antipsychotics with their serotonin/dopamine antagonism might induce *de novo* or aggravate preexisting OC symptoms in schizophrenia patients. Nevertheless, there is preliminary evidence indicating that monotherapy with some atypical antipsychotics may attenuate OC symptoms, pointing toward a potential bidirectional (alleviating vs. provoking) effect on OC symptoms in schizophrenia. Thus, olanzapine was efficacious in ameliorating both psychotic and OC symptoms in a large-scale randomized study in young patients with recent-onset schizophrenia-spectrum disorders.[71] By the end of a 6-week trial, olanzapine (mean dose 11.3 mg/day) but not risperidone (mean dose 3.0 mg/day) was associated with a meaningful decrease in the severity of OC symptoms (YBOCS, -2.2 vs.-0.3, z = -2.651, $P < .01$).

Similarly, in a 6-week, open-label, flexible-dose trial, monotherapy with aripiprazole (10–30 mg/day) resulted in a meaningful clinical improvement of OC symptoms in schizophrenia patients who were partially responsive to a prior exposure to either typical or atypical antipsychotic agents.[72] Even modest improvement of functioning, due to improvement in OC symptoms, as in this study, might be clinically meaningful for schizophrenia patients. In addition, amisulpride (not currently available in the United States) may effect amelioration of OC symptoms in schizophrenia patients.[73-75] Although the underlying mechanism of this positive effect of antipsychotics on OC symptoms is unclear, it could be related to differing serotonergic effects. Notably, aripiprazole is distinguished by its partial dopamine agonism coupled with a low 5-HT$_2$ to D$_2$ affinity ratio and a low 5-HT$_{1A}$ receptor occupancy.[76] Amisulpride is distinguished by its highly selective dopamine D$_2$/D$_3$ receptor antagonism and a minimal affinity for the 5-HT$_{2A}$ receptor.[77]

ADDITION OF SEROTONIN REUPTAKE INHIBITORS FOR OBSESSIVE-COMPULSIVE SCHIZOPHRENIA

The independent nature of OC symptoms in a vast majority of patients with OC-SCZ and their clinical similarity with "pure" OCD prompted evaluation of adjunctive anti-obsessive agents for antipsychotic-treated schizophrenia patients. Adjunctive escitalopram (10–40 mg/day), a common SSRI, showed a beneficial effect on OC symptoms in several open-label prospective trials in schizophrenia patients.[78,79] The drug's well-tolerated side effect profile and paucity of drug-drug interactions was substantiated. No clinically significant side effects or worsening of psychosis were observed.

On the other hand, while adjunctive fluvoxamine (100–200 mg/day) has been evaluated in several small studies and demonstrated its potential to reduce the severity of OC symptoms and associated pathologic slowness and doubt,[26,80] side effect concerns remain. Fluvoxamine may exacerbate psychosis and increase aggressiveness in those OC-SCZ patients with prior impulsivity or aggressive behavior.

Adjunctive clomipramine, a tricyclic antidepressant and a nonselective SRI, was also evaluated as a putative therapeutic option, but with important side effect concerns. A small placebo-controlled crossover study and a number of case reports revealed that clomipramine (dose range 50–300 mg/day) was associated with a beneficial effect on OC symptoms, reduction of anxiety accompanied by compulsive rituals, and improvement of positive and negative schizophrenia symptoms in some OC-SCZ patients.[81,82] However, lack of therapeutic effect of clomipramine and exacerbation of psychosis were also reported.[83] In addition, the anticholinergic properties of clomipramine, its cardiovascular side effects, and associated weight gain limit its utility in schizophrenia patients, particularly those who are treated with low-potency typical antipsychotic agents, anticholinergic agents, or clozapine.

Overall, the SSRIs exert a favorable effect on OC symptoms in certain schizophrenia patients. Therapeutic dose ranges for adjunctive SSRIs while treating schizophrenia patients are not well established. Indeed, a sizeable proportion of OC-SCZ patients do not respond or are intolerant to SSRI addition. Predictors of response and long-term treatment outcomes are not yet known. Limited clinical experience suggests that some OC-SCZ patients can better tolerate therapeutic SSRI doses if they also receive clonazepam q12h at an adequate dose.

An additional concern about of SSRI-antipsychotic drug combinations is the potential for clinically significant pharmacokinetic drug interactions. Fluvoxamine, fluoxetine, and paroxetine may elevate plasma concentrations of antipsychotics 2- to 10-fold.[84] This in turn may increase the likelihood of antipsychotic drug-induced side effects (e.g., extrapyramidal side effects, decreased seizure threshold, excessive sedation).

Clozapine is currently the most effective available antipsychotic. However, due to a high burden of adverse effects (e.g., potentially life-threatening agranulocytosis, paralytic ileus, seizures), clozapine is reserved for treatment-resistant schizophrenia patients. In contrast to apparent efficacy in schizophrenia patients, clozapine was found ineffective in patients with OCD.[85] There is compelling evidence that links clozapine with precipitating or worsening obsessions and compulsions in individuals with schizophrenia. However, there is also preliminary data indicating that clozapine in a relatively low-dose range with or without SSRIs may exert a beneficial effect at least in some OC-SCZ individuals.[26,86] Undoubtedly, more controlled investigations are warranted to elucidate predictors and risk factors of bidirectional (OC symptom-attenuating vs. OC symptom-provoking) effect of clozapine in patients with OC-SCZ.

Overall, it seems that for *some* patients with OC-SCZ, monotherapy with atypical antipsychotics may improve both schizophrenic and obsessive-compulsive dimensions of psychopathology without running the risk of OC symptom exacerbation. The identification of clinical and biological predictors of such a positive response is a major unmet need in pharmacologic management of patients with OC-SCZ.

NONPHARMACOLOGIC TREATMENT FOR OBSESSIVE-COMPULSIVE SCHIZOPHRENIA

Psychoeducation, stress management, and family support are important for patient management.[68,87] CBT along with pharmacotherapy is a first-line treatment for OCD. In contrast, the role of CBT in treating OC symptoms in schizophrenia is uncertain. This reflects concerns that accentuated stress of exposure-based interventions may increase vulnerability to psychotic relapse. Nevertheless, one open-label study reported that schizophrenia patients with OC symptoms do adhere to CBT, and that adjunctive CBT may be an effective alternative to an SSRI for at least some patients without increasing the risk of psychosis.[88]

On the positive side, CBT avoids drug-induced side effects and drug-drug interactions associated with adjunctive SSRIs, and may be beneficial to those where SSRIs are contraindicated or intolerable. Limitations include the need for an experienced therapist, cost, CBT treatment time span, and concerns about psychotogenic effects. A more graded approach for OC-SCZ patients than for patients with OCD alone seems reasonable. Close monitoring of mental state and regular assessments of symptoms are important for addressing all risks and benefits.

ELECTROCONVULSIVE THERAPY FOR OBSESSIVE-COMPULSIVE SCHIZOPHRENIA

Electroconvulsive therapy (ECT) is not an approved therapy for OCD. ECT is indicated for schizophrenia patients for catatonia, treatment resistance, and when pharmacotherapy is contraindicated. There are a few case reports that suggest the utility of ECT for patients with OC-SCZ who did not respond to or could not tolerate side effects associated with psychotropic agents and in cases in which the severity of the symptoms poses a serious threat to the patient's mental health and physical safety.[89,90] Side effects (e.g., memory disturbance), perceived stigma, and patient preference need to be considered prior to ECT.

TREATMENT OF OBSESSIVE-COMPULSIVE SYMPTOMS IN HIGH-RISK INDIVIDUALS

Pharmacotherapy should be considered, in addition to psychoeducation, family support, and stress management. SSRIs can be used for clinically significant OCD, combined with rigorous monitoring of attenuated positive symptoms. Some UHR patients with OCD/OC symptoms may benefit from a low-dose antipsychotic medication trial, even though these are not currently recommended for ongoing treatment of attenuated prodromal symptoms. Long-term treatment with antipsychotic agents should be considered only after the established diagnosis of schizophrenia. All treatment approaches require scrupulous risk/benefit evaluations.

ANTIPSYCHOTIC-INDUCED OBSESSIVE-COMPULSIVE SYMPTOMS

There are many reports that atypical antipsychotic agents with anti-serotonergic properties can induce or exacerbate OC symptoms.[74,91] While schizophrenia patients with preexisting OC symptoms may be at particular risk of drug-induced exacerbation of obsessions and compulsions, the majority of reports deal with *de novo* emergence of OC symptoms.

In most patients with olanzapine-, risperidone-, and quetiapine-induced OC symptoms, the symptoms appeared during initial treatment weeks. A wide dose range is associated with the OCD-provoking effects of olanzapine (5–25 mg/day) and clozapine (150–900 mg/day), but only relatively high risperidone (> 4 mg/day) and quetiapine (450–1100 mg/day).[92]

Dose reduction is a reasonable first step to control antipsychotic-induced OC symptoms.[52] A combination of a dose reduction and SSRI co-administration is an appropriate next step. Clomipramine may be needed to ameliorate antipsychotic-induced OC symptoms. Pharmacokinetic and pharmacodynamic drug-drug interactions should be explored carefully. Discontinuation of the offending compound and a switch to an atypical antipsychotic with lower potential to induce OC symptoms, such as aripiprazole and amisulpride, should be considered.[68]

Fictional Case: Prodromal Obsessive-Compulsive Disorder Preceding Schizophrenia Onset

A 28-year-old single white male began showing symptoms of OCD at age 12, including ritualistic touching before meals and prolonged handwashing many times each day. He was first brought to treatment at age 15, 7 months after he began to have paranoid delusions that his food had been poisoned, critical auditory hallucinations, and a slight reduction in obvious OC behaviors. He was diagnosed then with paranoid schizophrenia, and treated with a variety of antipsychotic medications over time. Each medication diminished but did not stop psychotic symptoms. He had several psychotic exacerbations over the years, each responding to temporarily increased antipsychotic medication.

His most recent hospitalization followed another acute exacerbation of paranoid delusion, auditory hallucinations with concurrent panic anxiety, accompanied by increased ritualistic behavior. In the hospital, he was noted as repetitively touching objects, opening and closing doors, and forcefully rubbing his eyes to the point of injury. Medical evaluation, including brain CT scan, was normal. His newly noted panic anxiety was treated with clonazepam titrated up to 1 mg q12h, while his newly diagnosed OCD was treated with fluoxetine, rapidly titrated up to 60 mg qd (clonazepam may have helped prevent potential fluoxetine-induced agitation). He was continued on fluphenazine decanoate (50 mg/2 weeks). After 4 weeks of fluoxetine 40 mg/day, his rituals became less frequent and intense, with improved socialization and therapy participation and a marked reduction in psychosis.

His family was happy with the level of improvement. Even so, there were brief episodes of noncompliance and ongoing non-psychotic emotional distress. Skillful psychotherapy was necessary to ensure medication compliance and to help him navigate the slow transition to a less symptomatic and more functional life.

Conclusions and future directions

Overall, a substantial body of evidence indicates that OCD and OC symptoms represent a clinically meaningful dimension of psychopathology in schizophrenia, and that OC-SCZ may have distinct clinical and neurobiological characteristics, treatment response, and prognosis, suggesting a possibly distinct diagnostic entity. Provisional diagnostic criteria for the identification of OC-SCZ have been suggested.[93]

Proposed Diagnostic Criteria for Obsessive-Compulsive Schizophrenia

(Schizophrenia With Obsessive-Compulsive Disorder)

A. Symptoms are present that meet Criterion A for obsessive-compulsive disorder at some time point during the course of the schizophrenia.
B. If the content of the obsessions and/or compulsions is interrelated with the content of delusions and/or hallucinations (e.g., compulsive handwashing due to command auditory hallucinations), additional typical OCD obsessions and compulsions recognized by the person as unreasonable and excessive are required.
C. Symptoms of obsessive-compulsive disorder are present for a substantial portion of the total duration of the prodromal, active, and/or residual period of schizophrenia.
D. The obsessions and compulsions are time consuming, cause distress, and significantly interfere with the person's normal routine, in addition to the functional impairment associated with schizophrenia.
E. The obsessions and compulsions in the patient with schizophrenia are not due to the direct effect of antipsychotic agents, a substance of abuse (e.g., cocaine), or an organic factor (e.g., head trauma).

Additional research is needed to delineate etiologic factors, neurobiology, psychopathology, and treatment of this OCD/OC symptom subset of schizophrenia patients. Large-scale studies should address diagnostic stability during long-term follow-up. Valid and reliable diagnostic instruments for assessing psychosis-related OC symptoms in schizophrenia patients, in addition to typical ego-dystonic OC symptoms, are needed. There may be distinct subgroups along a putative schizophrenia-OCD axis of disorders, including schizophrenia with OC symptoms versus primary OCD with poor insight or psychotic features.

Accurate diagnosis has prognostic and treatment implications. Current treatments for schizophrenia and OCD differ, and first-line medications for one disorder can exacerbate symptoms of the other: antipsychotics can exacerbate OC symptoms, and SSRIs may exacerbate psychosis. A search for effective, tolerable, and safe treatment that addresses both schizophrenic and OC symptoms in OC-SCZ patients is a central goal. Is fixed-dose clonazepam useful for preventing SSRI exacerbated psychosis?

Brain function studies can help ascertain whether OC symptoms modify patterns of brain activation in schizophrenia patients. A search for intermediate neurophysiologic and neurocognitive markers may also facilitate the delineation of an OC-SCZ subgroup. Further studies are essential to clarify whether the presence of OC symptoms in schizophrenia merely represents comorbidity of the two disorders or the distinct subtype of OC-SCZ.

References

1. American Psychiatric Association. *Diagnostic and Statistical Manual of Mental Disorders.* 5th ed. Arlington, VA: American Psychiatric Association; 2013.
2. Tandon R, Keshavan MS, Nasrallah HA. Schizophrenia "just the facts" what we know in 2008. *Epidemiol Etiol Schizoph Res.* 2008;102:1–18.
3. Andreasen NC. Thought, language, and communication disorders: I. Clinical assessment, definition of terms, and evaluation of their reliability. *Arch Gen Psychiatry.* 1979;36:1315–1321.
4. Andreasen NC. Negative symptoms in schizophrenia. Definition and reliability. *Arch Gen Psychiatry.* 1982;39:784–788.
5. Bloch MH, Landeros-Weisenberger A, Rosario MC, et al. Meta-analysis of the symptom structure of obsessive-compulsive disorder. *Am J Psychiatry.* 2008;165:1532–1542.
6. Amador XF, David AS, eds. *Insight and Psychosis.* New York: Oxford University Press; 1998.
7. Meier SM, Petersen L, Pedersen MG, et al. Obsessive-compulsive disorder as a risk factor for schizophrenia: a nationwide study. *JAMA Psychiatry.* 2014;71:1215–1221.
8. Cederlöf M, Lichtenstein P, Larsson H, et al. Obsessive-compulsive disorder, psychosis, and bipolarity: a longitudinal cohort and multigenerational family study. *Schizophr Bull.* 2015;41:1076–1083.
9. Yu-Fang C, Vincent C-H, Yao-Hsu Y, et al. Risk of schizophrenia among people with obsessive-compulsive disorder: a nationwide population-based cohort study. *Schizophr Res.* 2019;209:58–63.
10. Stengel EA. A study of some clinical aspects of the relationship between obsessional neurosis and psychotic reaction types. *J Ment Sci.* 1945;91:166–187.
11. Rosen I. The clinical significance of obsessions in schizophrenia. *J Ment Sci.* 1956;103:773–785.
12. Achim AM, Ouellet R, Roy MA, et al. Assessment of empathy in first-episode psychosis and meta-analytic comparison with previous studies in schizophrenia. *Psychiatry Res.* 2011;190:3–8.
13. Ruscio AM, Stein DJ, Chiu WT, et al. The epidemiology of obsessive-compulsive disorder in the National Comorbidity Survey Replication. *Mol Psychiatry.* 2010;15:53–63.
14. Porto L, Bermanzohn PC, Pollack S. A profile of obsessive-compulsive symptoms in schizophrenia. *CNS Spectr.* 1997;2:21–25.
15. Poyurovsky M, Weizman A, Weizman R. Obsessive-compulsive disorder in schizophrenia: clinical characteristics and treatment. *CNS Drugs.* 2004;18:989–1010.
16. Burgy M. Obsession in the strict sense: a helpful psychopathological phenomenon in the differential diagnosis between obsessive-compulsive disorder and schizophrenia. *PsychoPathology.* 2007;40:102–110.
17. Goodman WK, Price LH, Rasmussen SA, et al. The Yale-Brown Obsessive-Compulsive Scale. I. Development, use, and reliability. *Arch Gen Psychiatry.* 1989;46:1006–1011.
18. Tibbo P, Kroetsch M, Chue P, et al. Obsessive-compulsive disorder in schizophrenia. *J Psychiatr Res.* 2000;34(2):139–146.
19. Ongür D, Goff DC. Obsessive-compulsive symptoms in schizophrenia: associated clinical features, cognitive function and medication status. *Schizophr Res.* 2005;75(2–3):349–362.
20. Faragian S, Pashinian A, Fuchs C, et al. Obsessive-compulsive symptom dimensions in schizophrenia patients with comorbid obsessive-compulsive disorder. *Prog Neuropsychopharmacol Biol Psychiatry.* 2009;33(6):1009–1012.
21. de Haan L, Sterk B, Wouters L, et al. The 5-year course of obsessive-compulsive symptoms and obsessive-compulsive disorder in first-episode schizophrenia and related disorders. *Schizophr Bull.* 2013;39(1):151–160.
22 Poyurovsky M, Kriss V, Weisman G, et al. Comparison of clinical characteristics and comorbidity in schizophrenia patients with and without obsessive-compulsive disorder: schizophrenic and obsessive-compulsive symptoms in schizophrenia. *J Clin Psychiatry.* 2003;64(11):1300–1307.
23. Byerly M, Goodman W, Acholonu W, et al. Obsessive compulsive symptoms in schizophrenia: frequency and clinical features. *Schizophr Res.* 2005;76(2–3):309–316.
24. Hwang MY, Morgan JE, Losconzcy MF. Clinical and neuropsychological profiles of obsessive-compulsive schizophrenia: a pilot study. *J Neuropsychiatry Clin Neurosci.* 2000;12(1):91–94.
25. Ohta M, Kokai M, Morita Y. Features of obsessive-compulsive disorder in patients primarily diagnosed with schizophrenia. *Psychiatry Clin Neurosci.* 2003;57(1):67–74.
26. Poyurovsky M, Fuchs K, Weizman A. Obsessive-compulsive symptoms in patients with first episode schizophrenia. *Am J Psychiatry.* 1999;156:1998–2000.

27. de Haan L, Hoogeboom B, Beuk N, et al. Reliability and validity of the Yale-Brown Obsessive-Compulsive Scale in schizophrenia patients. *Psychopharmacol Bull.* 2006;39(1):25–30.
28. Rajkumar RP, Reddy YC, Kandavel T. Clinical profile of "schizo-obsessive" disorder: a comparative study. *Compr Psychiatry.* 2008;49(3):262–268.
29. Lysaker PH, Marks KA, Picone JB, et al. Obsessive and compulsive symptoms in schizophrenia: clinical and neurocognitive correlates. *J Nerv Ment Dis.* 2000;188(2):78–83.
30. Tiryaki A, Ozkorumak E. Do the obsessive-compulsive symptoms have an effect in schizophrenia? *Compr Psychiatry.* 2010;51(4):357–362. https://doi.org/10.1016/j.comppsych.2009.10.007.
31. Owashi T, Ota A, Otsubo T, et al. Obsessive-compulsive disorder and obsessive-compulsive symptoms in Japanese inpatients with chronic schizophrenia—a possible schizophrenic subtype. *Psychiatry Res.* 2010;179(3):241–246.
32. de Haan L, Hoogenboom B, Beuk N, et al. Obsessive-compulsive symptoms and positive, negative, and depressive symptoms in patients with recent-onset schizophrenic disorders. *Can J Psychiatry.* 2005;50(9):519–524.
33. Cunill R, Castells X, Simeon D. Relationships between obsessive-compulsive symptomatology and severity of psychosis in schizophrenia: a systematic review and meta-analysis. *J Clin Psychiatry.* 2009;70(1):70–82.
34. du Montcel C, Pelissolo A, Schürhoff F, et al. Obsessive-compulsive symptoms in schizophrenia: an up-to-date review of literature. *Curr Psychiatry Rep.* 2019;21(8):64.
35. Eisen JL, Rasmussen SA. Obsessive compulsive disorder with psychotic features. *J Clin Psychiatry.* 1993;54(10):373–379.
36. Kozak MJ, Foa EB. Obsessions, overvalued ideas, and delusions in obsessive-compulsive disorder. *Behav Res Ther.* 1994;32(3):343–353.
37. Amador XF, Flaum M, Andreasen NC, et al. Awareness of illness in schizophrenia and schizoaffective and mood disorders. *Arch Gen Psychiatry.* 1994;51(10):826–836.
38. Eisen JL, Phillips KA, Baer L, et al. The Brown Assessment of Beliefs Scale: reliability and validity. *Am J Psychiatry.* 1998;155(1):102–108.
39. Poyurovsky M, Faragian S, Kleinman-Balush V, et al. Awareness of illness and insight into obsessive-compulsive symptoms in schizophrenia patients with obsessive-compulsive disorder. *J Nerv Ment Dis.* 2007;195(9):765–768.
40. Tandon R, Nasrallah HA, Keshavan MS. Schizophrenia, "just the facts" 4. Clinical features and conceptualization. *Schizophr Res.* 2009;110:1–23.
41. Angermeyer K, Bermanzohn PC, Porto L, et al. Hierarchical diagnosis in chronic schizophrenia: a clinical study of co-occurring syndromes. *Schizophr Bull.* 2000;26:517–525.
42. Hafner H. The epidemiology of onset and course of schizophrenia. *Eur Arch Psychiatry Clin Neurosci.* 2000;250:292–303.
43. Ongur D, Lin L, Cohen BM. Clinical characteristics influencing age at onset in psychotic disorders. *Comprehens Psychiatry.* 2009;50:13–19.
44. Leckman JF, Denys D, Simpson HB, et al. Obsessive-compulsive disorder: a review of the diagnostic criteria and possible subtypes and dimensional specifiers for DSM-V. *Depress Anxiety.* 2010;27:507–527.
45. Brakoulias V, Starcevic V, Belloch A, et al. Comorbidity, age of onset and suicidality in obsessive-compulsive disorder (OCD): an international collaboration. *Compr Psychiatry.* 2017;76:79–86.
46. Devulapalli KK, Welge JA, Nasrallah HA. Temporal sequence of clinical manifestation in schizophrenia with comorbid OCD: review and meta-analysis. *Psychiatry Res.* 2008;161:105–108.
47. Faragian S, Fuchs CA, Weizman R, et al. Age-of-onset of schizophrenic and obsessive-compulsive symptoms in patients with schizo-obsessive disorder. *Psychiatry Res.* 2012;197(1–2):19–22.
48. Devi S, Rao NP, Badamath S, et al. Prevalence and clinical correlates of obsessive-compulsive disorder in schizophrenia. *Compr Psychiatry.* 2015;56:141–816.
49. Hwang MY, Kim S-W, Yum SY, et al. Management of schizophrenia with obsessive-compulsive features. *Psychiatry Clin North Am.* 2009;32:835–851.
50. Jaspers K. Basic philosophical writings. In: *The Collected Works.* Princeton, NJ: Princeton University Press; 1972.
51. Bermanzohn PC, Porto L, Arlow PB, Pollack S, Stronger R, Siris SG. Hierarchical diagnosis in chronic schizophrenia: a clinical study of co-occurring syndromes. *Schizophr Bull.* 2000;26(3):517–525.
52. Lykouras L, Alevizos B, Michalopoulou P, et al. Obsessive-compulsive symptoms induced by atypical antipsychotics. A review of the reported cases. *Prog Neuropsychopharmacol Biol Psychiatry.* 2003;27:333–346.

53. Szmulewicz AG, Smith JM, Valerio MP. Suicidality in clozapine-treated patients with schizophrenia: role of obsessive-compulsive symptoms. *Psychiatry Res.* 2015;230:50–55.

54. Hagen K, Hansen B, Joa I, et al. Prevalence and clinical characteristics of patients with obsessive-compulsive disorder in first-episode psychosis. *BMC Psychiatry.* 2013;13:156.

55. Addington D, Addington J, Maticka-Tyndale E, et al. Reliability and validity of a depression rating scale for schizophrenics. *Schizophr Res.* 1992;6(3):201–208.

56. Michalopoulou PG, Konstantakopoulos G, Typaldou M, et al. Can cognitive deficits differentiate between schizophrenia with and without obsessive-compulsive symptoms? *Compr Psychiatry.* 2014;55(4):1015–1021.

57. Nestadt G, Samuels J, Riddle MA, et al. The relationship between obsessive-compulsive disorder and anxiety and affective disorders: results from the Johns Hopkins OCD Family Study. *Psychol Med.* 2001;31(3):481–487.

58. Lochner C, Fineberg NA, Zohar J, et al. Comorbidity in obsessive-compulsive disorder (OCD): a report from the International College of Obsessive-Compulsive Spectrum Disorders (ICOCS). *Compr Psychiatry.* 2014;55:1513–1519.

59. Hollander E, Braun A, Simeon D. Should OCD leave the anxiety disorders in DSM-V? The case for obsessive compulsive-related disorders. *Depress Anxiety.* 2008;25(4):317–329. https://doi.org/10.1002/da.20500.

60. Phillips KA, Friedman MJ, Stein DJ, et al. Special DSM-V issues on anxiety, obsessive-compulsive spectrum, posttraumatic, and dissociative disorders. *Depress Anxiety.* 2010;27(2):91–92.

61. Poyurovsky M, Bergman J, Weizman R. Obsessive-compulsive disorder in elderly schizophrenia patients. *J Psychiatric Res.* 2006;40:189–191.

62. Nelson B, Yuen K, Yung AR. Ultra high risk (UHR) for psychosis criteria: are there different levels of risk for transition to psychosis? *Schizophr Res.* 2011;125:62–68.

63. Fusar-Poli P, Cappucciati M, Borgwardt S, et al. Heterogeneity of psychosis risk within individuals at clinical high risk: a meta-analytical stratification. *JAMA Psychiatry.* 2016;73:113–120.

64. Rosen JL, Miller TJ, D'Andrea JT, et al. Comorbid diagnoses in patients meeting criteria for the schizophrenia prodrome. *Schizophr Res.* 2006;85:124–131.

65. Niendam TA, Berzak J, Cannon TD, et al. Obsessive compulsive symptoms in the psychosis prodrome: correlates of clinical and functional outcome. *Schizophr Res.* 2009;108:170–175.

66. Fontenelle LF, Lin A, Pantelis C, et al. A longitudinal study of obsessive-compulsive disorder in individuals at ultra-high risk for psychosis. *J Psychiatr Res.* 2011;45:1140–1145.

67. Lencz T, Smith CW, Auther A, et al. Nonspecific and attenuated negative symptoms in patients at clinical high-risk for schizophrenia. *Schizophrenia Res.* 2004;68:37–48.

68. Zink M. Comorbid obsessive-compulsive symptoms in schizophrenia: insight into pathomechanisms facilitates treatment. *Adv Med.* 2014;2014:317980.

69. Mittal VA, Karlsgodt K, Zinberg J, et al. Identification and treatment of a pineal region tumor in an adolescent with prodromal psychotic symptoms. *Am J Psychiatry.* 2010;167(9):1033–1037.

70. Green AI, Canuso CM, Brenner MJ, et al. Detection and management of comorbidity in patients with schizophrenia. *Psychiatr Clin North Am.* 2003;26(1):115–139.

71. van Nimwegen L, de Haan L, van Beveren N, et al. Obsessive-compulsive symptoms in a randomized, double-blind study with olanzapine or risperidone in young patients with early psychosis. *J Clin Psychopharmacol.* 2008;28(2):214–218.

72. Glick ID, Poyurovsky M, Ivanova O, et al. Aripiprazole in schizophrenia patients with comorbid obsessive-compulsive symptoms: an open-label study of 15 patients. *J Clin Psychiatry.* 2008;69(12):1856–1859.

73. Kim SW, Shin IS, Kim JM, et al. Amisulpride improves obsessive-compulsive symptoms in schizophrenia patients taking atypical antipsychotics: an open-label switch study. *J Clin Psychopharmacol.* 2008;28:349–352.

74. Kim SW, Shin IS, Kim JM, et al. The 5-HT2 receptor profiles of antipsychotics in the pathogenesis of obsessive-compulsive symptoms in schizophrenia. *Clin Neuropharmacol.* 2009;32:224–226.

75. Schirmbeck F, Rausch F, Englisch S, et al. Differential effects of antipsychotic agents on obsessive-compulsive symptoms in schizophrenia: a longitudinal study. *J Psychopharmacol.* 2013;27(4):349–357.

76. Mamo D, Graff A, Mizrahi R, et al. Differential effects of aripiprazole on D(2), 5-HT(2), and 5-HT(1A) receptor occupancy in patients with schizophrenia: a triple tracer PET study. *Am J Psychiatry.* 2007;164(9):1411–1417.

77. Lecrubier Y, Azorin M, Bottai T, et al. Consensus on the practical use of amisulpride, an atypical antipsychotic, in the treatment of schizophrenia. *Neuropsychobiology.* 2001;44(1):41–46.
78. Stryjer R, Dambinsky Y, Timinsky I, et al. Escitalopram in the treatment of patients with schizophrenia and obsessive-compulsive disorder: an open-label, prospective study. *Int Clin Psychopharmacol.* 2013;28(2):96–98.
79. Rubin-Kahana DS, Shelef A, Weizman A, et al. The effectiveness of high-dose escitalopram in the treatment of patients suffering from schizophrenia with comorbid obsessive-compulsive disorder: an open-label study. *Int Clin Psychopharmacol.* 2019;34(4):179–183.
80. Reznik I, Sirota P. An open study of fluvoxamine augmentation of neuroleptics in schizophrenia with obsessive and compulsive symptoms. *Clin Neuropharmacol.* 2000;23(3):157–160.
81. Zohar J, Kaplan Z, Benjamin J. Clomipramine treatment of obsessive compulsive symptomatology in schizophrenic patients. *J Clin Psychiatry.* 1993;54(10):385–388.
82. Berman I, Sapers BL, Chang HH, et al. Treatment of obsessive-compulsive symptoms in schizophrenic patients with clomipramine. *J Clin Psychopharmacol.* 1995;15(3):206–210.
83. Margetić B, Aukst-Margetić B, Jakovljević M. Aggravation of schizophrenia by clomipramine in a patient with comorbid obsessive-compulsive disorder. *Psychopharmacol Bull.* 2008;41(2):9–11.
84. Hiemke C, Weigmann H, Härtter S, et al. Elevated levels of clozapine in serum after addition of fluvoxamine. *J Clin Psychopharmacol.* 1994;14(4):279–281.
85. McDougle CJ, Barr LC, Goodman WK, et al. Lack of efficacy of clozapine monotherapy in refractory obsessive-compulsive disorder. *Am J Psychiatry.* 1995;152(12):1812–1814.
86. Tibbo P, Gendemann K. Improvement of obsessions and compulsions with clozapine in an individual with schizophrenia. *Can J Psychiatry.* 1999;44(10):1049–1050.
87. Haroun N, Dunn L, Haroun A, et al. Risk and protection in prodromal schizophrenia: ethical implications for clinical practice and future research. *Schizophr Bull.* 2006;32(1):166–178.
88. Tundo A, Salvati L, Di Spigno D, et al. Cognitive-behavioral therapy for obsessive-compulsive disorder as a comorbidity with schizophrenia or schizoaffective disorder. *Psychother Psychosom.* 2012;81(1):58–60.
89. Hanisch F, Friedemann J, Piro J, et al. Maintenance electroconvulsive therapy for comorbid pharmacotherapy-refractory obsessive-compulsive and schizoaffective disorder. *Eur J Med Res.* 2009;14(8):367–368.
90. Rao NP, Antony A, Raveendranathan D, et al. Successful use of maintenance electroconvulsive therapy in the treatment of clozapine-associated obsessive-compulsive symptoms in schizophrenia: a case report. *J ECT.* 2011;27(1):e37–e38.
91. Sharma LP, Reddy YCJ. Obsessive-compulsive disorder comorbid with schizophrenia and bipolar disorder. *Indian J Psychiatry.* 2019;61(Suppl 1):S140–S148.
92. Chen CH, Chiu CC, Huang MC. Dose-related exacerbation of obsessive-compulsive symptoms with quetiapine treatment. *Prog Neuropsychopharmacol Biol Psychiatry.* 2008 1;32(1):304–305.
93. Poyurovsky M. *Schizo-Obsessive Disorder.* Cambridge: Cambridge University Press; 2013.

CHAPTER 4

Paranoid Schizophrenia With Voices and Panic Anxiety

Jeffrey Paul Kahn

Abstract

Panic anxiety may be the most common specific subtype of anxiety. It can appear at an early age as separation anxiety, and return in adolescence in situations of real or symbolic separation. It is generally chronic, variably intense, and with characteristic episodes of paroxysmal panic anxiety. DSM-5 requires the paroxysmal panic to be accompanied by at least four of certain physical and cognitive symptoms. Accurate diagnosis requires a focused interview segment that explores internal experience, as panics are rarely obvious to observers. Ongoing anticipatory anxiety is common, and may be misread as generalized anxiety. Schizophrenia is a chronic progressive illness that includes both positive psychotic symptoms as well as negative social withdrawal symptoms. Studies have suggested a high comorbidity of panic and schizophrenia, and some evidence suggests that most schizophrenia patients with auditory hallucinations may have panic anxiety manifesting in psychotic form as voices. Medications for treatment of psychosis do not eliminate risk and consequences of panic anxiety. Careful diagnosis of both conditions is important for optimal outcomes. Augmentation with fixed-dose q12h clonazepam is often beneficial in patients with voices, after careful attention to potential risks and benefits. Various lines of emerging evidence suggest the possibility of a panic psychosis.

KEYWORDS

Panic   Anxiety   Psychosis   Hallucination   Schizophrenia

This volume makes the point that every patient with psychosis requires a careful differential diagnosis, and that there is more to diagnosis than just the monolithic concept of "schizophrenia." Moreover, the ancillary anxiety and depressive symptoms of psychotic disorders are not just "understandable" artifacts of a distressing disease. For example, DSM-5 notes that "anxiety and phobias are common" in schizophrenia.[1] But it could well be that five specific anxiety and depressive subtype syndromes may be the core of five corresponding psychotic disorders, and they may be the key to understanding and categorizing discrete psychosis subtypes. Each one requires careful and informed clinical evaluation, each has its own phenomenology and prognosis, and each has a specific treatment approach that can be much more effective than antipsychotic medications alone.

The idea that comorbid syndromes could play a central role in psychotogenesis goes back more than 100 years.[2] Early observers tended to view anxiety as a predecessor and contributor to schizophrenia, although more recent scholars have been more likely to consider anxiety and depression as comorbid syndromes that may result from schizophrenia.

Schizophrenia

Of the five core comorbidity syndromes in this book, the one that looks much like classic paranoid schizophrenia with auditory hallucinations is schizophrenia with comorbid panic anxiety. Indeed, the name "Panic Psychosis" has been proposed for this syndrome.[3] In addition, there can be other psychosis comorbidities such as obsessive-compulsive disorder (Chapter 3) and social anxiety disorder (Chapter 5; focusing primarily on Persecutory Delusional disorder).

Schizophrenia is defined in DSM-5[1] (Table 4.1).

When viewed as a single entity, lifetime schizophrenia prevalence is estimated at 0.7%.[4] It is important to remember that schizophrenia diagnosis requires at least 6 sustained months of illness. Shorter durations with similar symptoms include brief reactive psychosis and schizophreniform disorder, and do not necessarily progress to schizophrenia. Importantly, the differential diagnosis includes delusional disorder (Chapter 5), psychotic depression (Chapter 6), bipolar psychosis (Chapter 7), substance-induced psychosis (Chapter 8), medical illness and iatrogenic psychosis (Chapter 9), as well as the concepts of schizo-obsessive disorder (Chapter 3) and the panic psychosis discussed in this chapter.

TABLE 4.1 ■ **Diagnostic Criteria: Schizophrenia**

DSM-5: 295.90 (ICD10: F20.9)

A. Two (or more) of the following, each present for a significant portion of time during a 1-month period (or less if successfully treated). At least one of these must be (1), (2), or (3):
  1. Delusions.
  2. Hallucinations.
  3. Disorganized speech (e.g., frequent derailment or incoherence).
  4. Grossly disorganized or catatonic behavior.
  5. Negative symptoms (i.e., diminished emotional expression or avolition).

B. For a significant portion of the time since the onset of the disturbance, level of functioning in one or more major areas, such as work, interpersonal relations, or self-care, is markedly below the level achieved prior to the onset (or when the onset is in childhood or adolescence, there is failure to achieve expected level of interpersonal, academic, or occupational functioning).

C. Continuous signs of the disturbance persist for at least 6 months. This 6-month period must include at least 1 month of symptoms (or less if successfully treated) that meet Criterion A (i.e., active-phase symptoms) and may include periods of prodromal or residual symptoms. During these prodromal or residual periods, the signs of the disturbance may be manifested by only negative symptoms or by two or more symptoms listed in Criterion A present in an attenuated form (e.g., odd beliefs, unusual perceptual experiences).

D. Schizoaffective disorder and depressive or bipolar disorder with psychotic features have been ruled out because either (1) no major depressive or manic episodes have occurred concurrently with the active-phase symptoms or (2) if mood episodes have occurred during active-phase symptoms, they have been present for a minority of the total duration of the active and residual periods of the illness.

E. The disturbance is not attributable to the physiologic effects of a substance (e.g., a drug of abuse, a medication) or another medical condition.

F. If there is a history of autism spectrum disorder or a communication disorder of childhood onset, the additional diagnosis of schizophrenia is made only if prominent delusions or hallucinations, in addition to the other required symptoms of schizophrenia, are also present for at least 1 month (or less if successfully treated).

Schizophrenia (page 87—code 295.90, F20).
American Psychiatric Association. Schizophrenia spectrum and other psychotic disorders. In *Diagnostic and statistical Manual of Mental Disorders*. 5th ed. 2013. https://doi.org/10.1176/appi.books.9780890425596. dsm02.

Recent research has suggested that there may be a genetically influenced susceptibility to schizophrenia underlying five distinct subtypes of schizophrenia. Two studies each used factor analysis of common symptoms to propose their similar five subtypes.[5,6] On the surface, there is some suggestion that they may correspond with the same five psychoses previously proposed clinically,[7] documented in a small pilot study of schizophrenia comorbidity subtype diagnosis,[8] and now considered here (along with substance and medically related psychoses).

Schizophrenia is a chronic, progressive, and debilitating disease. Symptoms are typically grouped into positive psychotic symptoms and negative social symptoms. The positive symptoms can include auditory hallucinations, paranoid delusions, and ideas of reference. Ideas of reference include self-referential belief that there are special personal meanings in radio or television broadcasts, glances or sounds from strangers, or in news events. Negative symptoms can include apathy and limitations in affective display, speech output, social interaction, capacity for pleasure, and motivation. Schizophrenia symptoms produce substantial social and cognitive limitations. With onset typically in adolescence or early adulthood, education and social development are seriously disrupted, and the disruption typically continues even with decent response to antipsychotic medications.[2]

These medications can reduce psychosis and rehospitalization, but schizophrenia remains a life-changing illness. To be sure, some people do return to a more normal life and function, and some may even experience substantially full recovery.[2] But research and anecdotal evidence presented in this volume suggest that the degree and duration of improvement can be substantially increased with diagnosis and treatment of comorbid, and perhaps underlying, psychiatric disorders.

There are financial costs to society as well. Schizophrenia impairs occupational and social function, contributes to homelessness, and to needs for external family, community, and financial support. There is also a significant cost of medical and psychiatric care. Any increased cost of improved diagnosis and treatment would be offset by reductions in some of these other costs, not to mention the personal, familial, and societal benefits.

Panic Disorder

This chapter focuses on comorbidity of panic disorder with schizophrenia, panic exacerbation of schizophrenia, and the proposed notion of a panic psychosis. Panic disorder is defined in DSM-5[1] (Table 4.2).

Panic disorder (panic anxiety) diagnosis requires a specific and detailed clinical inquiry about paroxysmal onset episodes of panic anxiety, and about related symptoms. For example, panic underlies most phobias, and is often associated with chronic anticipatory anxiety (commonly experienced as generalized anxiety). Anticipatory anxiety is understood as ongoing non-panic anxiety unwittingly caused by fearful uncertainty about when the next panic will occur. Research suggests that a significant percentage of those with generalized anxiety disorder have underlying but unrecognized panic disorder.

Panic attacks can't be quantified by clinician observation, as only rarely are they outwardly visible to other people. Until diagnosis, people with panic attacks often experience them as merely an escalation of anxiety, rather than as a discrete and paroxysmal subtype of anxiety. In addition, they often attribute panics to being trapped, and thus unable to escape from some kind of physical danger. The perceived danger can also be related to actual panic symptoms, and so lead people to other physicians before psychiatrists. For example, chest pain can lead to concerns about heart attacks, shortness of breath to asthma, and other symptoms to many more medical concerns. After diagnosis, patients become more able to experience panics as internally generated, as discrete episodes, and often in response to some known or unknown symbolic emotional threat.

Panic disorder is common in the general population, with an estimated US population prevalence of 4.8%.[9] It is generally thought that most people are not able to panic, even in response to

TABLE 4.2 ■ Diagnostic Criteria: Panic Disorder

DSM-5: 300.01 (ICD10: F41.0)

A. Recurrent unexpected panic attacks. A panic attack is an abrupt surge of intense fear or intense discomfort that reaches a peak within minutes, and during which time four (or more) of the following symptoms occur:
   Note: The abrupt surge can occur from a calm state or an anxious state.
   1. Palpitations, pounding heart, or accelerated heart rate.
   2. Sweating.
   3. Trembling or shaking.
   4. Sensations of shortness of breath or smothering.
   5. Feelings of choking.
   6. Chest pain or discomfort.
   7. Nausea or abdominal distress.
   8. Feeling dizzy, unsteady, light-headed, or faint.
   9. Chills or heat sensations.
   10. Paresthesias (numbness or tingling sensations).
   11. Derealization (feelings of unreality) or depersonalization (being detached from oneself).
   12. Fear of losing control or "going crazy."
   13. Fear of dying.
   Note: Culture-specific symptoms (e.g., tinnitus, neck soreness, headache, uncontrollable screaming or crying) may be seen. Such symptoms should not count as one of the four required symptoms.

B. At least one of the attacks has been followed by 1 month (or more) of one or both of the following:
   1. Persistent concern or worry about additional panic attacks or their consequences (e.g., losing control, having a heart attack, "going crazy").
   2. A significant maladaptive change in behavior related to the attacks (e.g., behaviors designed to avoid having panic attacks, such as avoidance of exercise or unfamiliar situations).

C. The disturbance is not attributable to the physiologic effects of a substance (e.g., a drug of abuse, a medication) or another medical condition (e.g., hyperthyroidism, cardiopulmonary disorders).

D. The disturbance is not better explained by another mental disorder (e.g., the panic attacks do not occur only in response to feared social situations, as in social anxiety disorder; in response to circumscribed phobic objects or situations, as in specific phobia; in response to obsessions, as in obsessive-compulsive disorder; in response to reminders of traumatic events, as in posttraumatic stress disorder; or in response to separation from attachment figures, as in separation anxiety disorder).

Panic Disorder (page 208—code 300.01, F41).
American Psychiatric Association. Anxiety disorders. In *Diagnostic and Statistical Manual of Mental Disorders*. 5th ed. 2013. https://doi.org/10.1176/appi.books.9780890425596.dsm05

laboratory challenge procedures known to provoke panic in people who have the syndrome. So, if you include all those people who report even one lifetime panic attack, the population prevalence for panic susceptibility may be closer to 23%. Even in a large sample of corporate employees, the lifetime prevalence of at least one panic attack was 15%, disproportionately occurring in lower-level job categories.[10]

Panic disorder typically begins in early to mid-adolescence, but is sometimes preceded by an earlier period of separation anxiety in toddlers. Individual panic attacks typically last for several minutes, but can last for hours or even days. Prolonged panic attacks contribute to agitation and agitated behavior.[11] Untreated, panic disorder symptom severity waxes and wanes over a lifetime, frequently with lengthy panic-free periods, and often with development of coping skills that reduce some of the emotional and functional impediments to social and occupational accomplishment. Panic is also a predictive risk factor for some medical diagnoses, including heart disease and stroke.

Psychosis-Like Symptoms in Non-Psychotic Panic Disorder

Two studies have reported that ideas of reference and paranoid ideation, drawn from the psychoticism and paranoia subscales of the SCL-90, were significantly more common in panic patients with no psychosis history than in no-panic controls.[12,13] These same symptoms are also among those considered markers for psychosis-proneness.

Schizophrenia with Auditory Hallucinations and Comorbid Panic

Many studies have noted a high prevalence of comorbid panic anxiety in schizophrenia. In the Epidemiological Catchment Area study (ECA), 45% of schizophrenia patients had a lifetime history of panic attacks.[14,15] In one small sample of patients with schizophrenia with voices, 100% had panic associated with their voices, as well as carbon dioxide challenge test induced panic.[16] Many other studies have reported a significantly increased panic prevalence rate in schizophrenia. Where there is variation in prevalence rate, it may be due to different methods for panic diagnosis, less specific criteria for schizophrenia diagnosis (i.e., sometimes including other psychotic disorders), the difficulty of diagnosing panic when it appears in psychotic form,[17] or when cognitive impairment clouds awareness.[18] Panic, like the other comorbidities in this volume, is easiest to diagnose when psychotic patients have been stabilized, and by including a careful history of panic that preceded psychosis onset. Importantly, an earlier history of prodromal panics suggests ongoing chronic panic disorder, or at least chronic susceptibility.

Compared to other schizophrenia patients, comorbid panic and schizophrenia is associated with earlier age of onset, more severe illness course, more severe symptoms, more positive psychotic symptoms, more paranoid features, more suicidal thought, and lower quality of life.[14,15,19–22]

Panic can itself appear in psychotic form, notably as auditory hallucinations, but also as acutely exacerbated paranoid delusions.[23] As noted below, specific interview techniques are essential for evaluating these possibilities. This approach is used by the semi-structured Panic and Schizophrenia Interview (PaSI). In two small PaSI studies, the voices also met DSM panic criteria in 73% and in 100% of patients.[8,16] In the second of those studies, PaSI interview findings were confirmed in the laboratory by a randomized and blinded carbon dioxide panic challenge test. Carbon dioxide provoked panic in all eight subjects, while placebo provoked panic in only one. Not surprisingly, some patients describe more panic attacks when they become non-hallucinatory.[24] At that point, many patients will understand the concept of their now ordinary panic attacks as "voices without the voices." Consistent with the notion of ongoing anticipatory anxiety in ordinary panic, some patients with voices experience ongoing paranoid fears about the recurrently frightening characters and messages in their voices.

Recent research on both panic and schizophrenia has looked at pathophysiology of the GABA neurotransmitter system, prefrontal cortex function, and at genetic and familial observations. To start, one study has shown that unselected schizophrenia patients, as compared to controls, have a nearly five times higher prevalence of panic disorder among their first-degree relatives.[25] When healthy relatives of schizophrenia patients were given low-dose alprazolam, they had a distinctive GABA response as compared to healthy relatives of normal controls.[26] The GABA neurotransmitter system regulates anxiety, with different GABA receptor subtypes influencing varied anxiety subtypes. In general, reduced GABA activity is associated with increased anxiety. Not surprisingly, genetic research shows that panic disorder is associated with GABRA5 (alpha 5 receptor subunits) and GABRB3 (beta 3 receptor subunits) genes and associated dysfunction.[27]

Similarly, panic disorder patients have decreased GABA levels in the prefrontal cortex.[28] Another study showed reduced GABA receptor binding in the prefrontal cortex (primary site of conscious thought), which correlated with panic symptom severity.[29]

Schizophrenia research similarly suggests deficient GABA activity in the prefrontal cortex.[30] A study of first-episode patients found comparable results, along with compensatory increased glutamate activity.[31] Schizophrenia patients with reduced prefrontal cortex size (associated with psychosis susceptibility) had a stronger clinical response to alprazolam.[32] While much research is still needed, these paired panic and schizophrenia findings suggest that some specific form of deficient GABAergic transmission could be an underlying mechanism that connects panic with some schizophrenia.[33] Clonazepam, or similarly acting present and future medications, may help by acting on this shared mechanism.

Fictional Case

Helen, an 18-year-old high school graduate from Texas, began feeling more anxious at age 14, especially when she was away from home and family. At first, she just thought this was just occasional distress about going to school, or about getting stuck in traffic jams. But soon the anxiety became more constant, though with varying intensity. Grades and social life began to suffer. At 16, Helen's parents brought her for counseling. She learned helpful techniques for understanding and coping with the anxiety, but it did not go away. She also came to realize that the worst part of the anxiety came on as very sudden panic, with sweating, an urge to flee, racing heart, shakiness, shortness of breath, and a fear that something dreadful would happen.

At 18, she began to hear a voice talking to her. The voice would also begin very suddenly, together with her other panic symptoms. This harsh and critical voice was quite real to her, and far more troubling than the other symptoms. She found it increasingly hard to motivate herself, to enjoy anything, or to socialize. After some months of increasingly paranoid fears, social withdrawal, and emotional detachment, she was brought to see a psychiatrist.

Evaluation included careful psychiatric history from Helen and family, medical consultation, evaluation of possible substance abuse and suicide risk, and consideration of elective hospitalization. At first, her acute psychosis was treated as an outpatient with risperidone, and after a month (6 months from illness onset) she had a significant reduction in her voices and paranoid fears. At that point, the psychiatrist reviewed her psychosis history and her potential comorbid and premorbid symptoms. Helen was newly able to recall and describe the panic attacks that had started at 14. When asked, she was also able to describe the paroxysmal onset of her auditory hallucination episodes, and how they were accompanied by the same sudden symptoms as her panic attacks. Now that the voices were far less common, she also began to notice the return of panic attacks without voices. Other common comorbidities were not present.

Helen's risperidone was augmented with clonazepam q12h fixed dose (no PRNs). Medications were given by her family, and the initial clonazepam dose was small. She was warned that she might feel drowsy for a few days each time the clonazepam dose was raised. Over the course of a few weeks, her dose was slowly raised to the point where even mild voices and panics had fully ceased at 2 mg q12h. The paranoid fears steadily faded in importance. Helen remembered them only when asked, and they were of rather little concern. Little or no drowsiness remained. Ironically, as she reached the point where her symptoms were essentially gone, she became quite concerned about medication side effects, and wanted to stop treatment. This concern was addressed in psychotherapy by carefully explaining the difference between illness and treatment. Therapy also discussed her dread of a serious illness, as well as her uncertainty about the likelihood of continuing to feel well.

Feeling her best since age 14, Helen was soon able to start college. She remained in weekly therapy with a local psychiatrist, established a social network, and did well in class. After a year or so, her risperidone dose was reduced. Three years later, fully compliant with treatment, she continued to do well, and was hopeful for the future.

Interview Technique

A skilled interview requires clinical training and expert familiarity with schizophrenia and panic diagnostic criteria and phenomenology. The detailed assessment below is typically more effective after acute psychosis is already stabilized. Some basic guidelines for interviewing psychotic patients are included in Chapter 1. After establishing a diagnostic alliance with the patient, ask patients if there are times when they are not actively hearing voices. Then ask if, at least sometimes, the voices return with a paroxysmal onset (regardless of any reported triggering events at those moments). While repeatedly focusing on that paroxysmal moment, ask about concurrent panic, fear, or anxiety, as well as the other DSM-5 panic symptoms. A detailed semi-structured clinical approach to DSM-5 panic diagnosis in schizophrenia is included in the PaSI, intended as a supplement to a full psychiatric history. Like any diagnostic interview, the sensitivity and specificity of diagnostic data may be limited by clinicians' experience, and by patients' cognitive impairment, personality, and fearfulness. Since the PaSI focuses on careful evaluation of psychotic symptoms for concurrent panic symptoms, this part of the clinical interview may need 15 minutes to complete.

Panic and Schizophrenia Interview

Let's talk for a minute about your voices.

[IDENTIFYING PAROXYSMAL MOMENTS OF VOICE ONSET]
Do you hear voices at every single moment, or are they sometimes silent?
Think about those times when you are not actually hearing any voices.
Now, there may be reasons why the voices start talking when they do, but let's leave that aside for now.
So, whenever the voices do begin speaking—and for whatever reason they do—is it all of a sudden, or do they start very softly and then very gradually get louder?
If your voices are nearly always there, then are there times when the voices suddenly come back, get louder, get more insistent, or just get more obvious to you?

[FOCUS PATIENT ON SUDDEN MOMENT OF VOICE ONSET, INTENSIFICATION, OR AWARENESS]
Let's talk about that sudden moment when the voices begin (or intensify, or become obvious), even if you know the reason why they start.
I'm going to ask you about some symptoms that you might have at that same sudden moment when the voices start (or intensify, or become obvious).
If you have any of these symptoms at the other times, they do not count for now.
So, when I ask about each symptom, tell me whether it comes on at the same sudden moments as the voices, and also if it used to come on with the voices in the past.
For each sudden symptom just say "YES" or "NO" or "SOMETIMES."

[FREQUENTLY SUBSTITUTE: "AT THE SAME SUDDEN MOMENTS THAT THE VOICES COME ON"]

1.	Sudden anxiety, fear, or panic on the inside?		Y	N	S
2.	Sudden anger or rage on the inside?	[ANGER QUERY]	Y	N	S
3.	Sudden heart racing? Heart pounding?		Y	N	S
4.	Sudden chest pain? Chest pressure?		Y	N	S
5.	Sudden sweating?		Y	N	S
6.	Sudden trembling or shaking?		Y	N	S
7.	Sudden shortness of breath, or like you can't catch your breath?		Y	N	S
8.	Sudden choking or a lump in your throat?		Y	N	S
9.	Sudden nausea or queasiness?		Y	N	S
10.	Sudden dizziness, lightheadedness, or faintness?		Y	N	S
11.	Sudden feeling of detachment, sort of like you are in a glass box?		Y	N	S
12.	Sudden fear of losing control? Fear of going crazy?		Y	N	S
13.	Sudden fear afraid of dying? Afraid of having a heart attack?		Y	N	S

(Continued)

Panic and Schizophrenia Interview—cont'd

14.	Sudden numbness or tingling, especially in your hands or face?		Y	N	S
15.	Sudden feeling of heat, or cold?		Y	N	S
16.	Sudden itching in your teeth?	[VALIDITY CHECK]	Y	N	S
17.	Sudden fear that people want to hurt you?	[EXCESS FEAR QUERY]	Y	N	S
18.	Sudden voices?	[VOICES QUERY]	Y	N	S

[PAST & PRODROMAL PANIC HISTORY]

At what age did you first see a therapist or psychiatrist?   _____

At what age were you first hospitalized for an emotional problem?   _____

At what age did you first start hearing voices?   _____

At what age did you first start having strong fears of other people?   _____

Before you ever heard voices, did you ever have any of the other sudden symptoms like the ones we just talked about?	(Yes/No/ Maybe)	Y N M	
Did those episodes back then feel sort of like your voices or sudden fears do now, except that there were no voices or sudden fears of people back then?		Y N M	

At what age did those sudden anxiety (or panic or rage) episodes begin?   _____

Back then, did you feel MORE sudden anxiety, or the SAME amount of sudden anxiety, or LESS sudden anxiety than you do now with your sudden voices?   M   S   L

[PAST & PRODROMAL PANIC SYMPTOMS]
Now let's talk about some symptoms that you might have had at those same sudden anxiety moments, in the time before you ever heard any voices.
So, for each sudden symptom just say "YES" or "NO" or "SOMETIMES."

[FREQUENTLY SUBSTITUTE: "AT THE SAME MOMENT THE SUDDEN ANXIETY CAME ON—

BUT ONLY DURING THE TIME BEFORE YOU EVER HEARD SUDDEN VOICES"]

[ASK ABOUT THE SAME 18 PANIC-RELATED SYMPTOMS LISTED ABOVE]

[PHOBIA-RELATED PANIC AND VOICES]

Have you ever been afraid to go into a (car, bus, plane, train, subway, elevator, mall, tunnel, bridge, heights, small place, CAT scan or MRI, being alone, crowds)?   Y   N   M

[IF YES OR MAYBE, PANIC SYMPTOMS IN PHOBIC SITUATIONS]
Now let's talk about some symptoms that you might have had at some of those times you were afraid.
So, for each symptom just say "YES" or "NO" or "SOMETIMES."

[ASK ABOUT THE SAME 18 PANIC-RELATED SYMPTOMS LISTED ABOVE]

At what age did you last have sudden anxiety without voices?   _____

Has medication ever completely stopped your voices? Somewhat?   Y   N   M

If so, did those other sudden symptoms still happen sometimes?   Y   N   M

Thank you for your help, and for answering all these questions!
PaSI © Jeffrey P Kahn MD

Treatment

Effective treatment of comorbid paranoid schizophrenia with voices and panic disorder starts with accurate diagnosis, and consideration of other possible comorbidities. It is not uncommon to have more than one comorbidity with a psychotic disorder, and all may require appropriate treatment. For panic as a sole comorbidity, it is often necessary to stabilize the psychosis before a complete and accurate history can be obtained. Clinical experience suggests that clonazepam q12h adjunctive to conventional antipsychotic medication can improve acute treatment of schizophrenia with voices. An open study of schizophrenia and panic showed a consistent and marked improvement in all seven inpatients treated with adjunctive alprazolam, and a return of symptoms when alprazolam was tapered.[34] This is also supported by one randomized study of alprazolam for agitated schizophrenia ER patients (not all with voices).[35] Alprazolam and clonazepam are the two benzodiazepines approved and effective for panic, but alprazolam is more problematic in clinical practice.

Once panics are identified, typically as concurrent symptoms of paroxysmal voices, clonazepam q12h fixed dose (no PRNs) can be started, with both voices and panics as target symptoms. Raising the dose gradually has the three advantages of allowing tolerance to initial sedative effects, allowing patients time to adjust to clinical improvement by effecting gradual improvement, and arriving at the lowest fully effective dose of clonazepam. For treatment of ordinary panic, one estimate of final clonazepam dose range is between 2 and 5 mg/day for most patients (divided into q12h or q8h fixed doses; no PRNs), and may be slightly less if concurrent with an SSRI.[36] Doses are likely similar for panic comorbid with schizophrenia although full cessation of panic and voices may rarely require slightly more.

Paranoid delusions will decrease in intensity over time, and gradually become unimportant to the patient, though sometimes still faintly believed. Clonazepam (and alprazolam) may allow lower initial and maintenance neuroleptic doses. Over an extended (though yet undefined) time period, it may be possible to reduce antipsychotic doses.[37] This can sometimes be done after a year, and may reduce risk of long-term antipsychotic side effects. Clonazepam doses may continue unchanged for an extended period of time.

Clonazepam is not the only anti-panic medication, but is highly effective in proper dose, and has a long enough half-life that q12h dosing is usually sufficient. Although alprazolam is similarly effective,[34] its shorter half-life means that stable blood levels are more difficult to achieve, and alprazolam also has a higher abuse potential. Tricyclic antidepressants were the first known anti-panic medication, and can be highly effective for ordinary panic. In psychosis, however, there is as yet no good evidence that they contribute to antipsychotic benefit, and may even worsen psychosis in some cases. SSRIs and SNRIs are commonly used for ordinary panic, but may be less effective, and as yet have little evidence for adjunctive anti-psychotic benefit. SSRIs may be useful, though, as adjuncts for schizophrenia comorbid with obsessive-compulsive disorder (OCD) (Chapter 3) and social anxiety (Chapter 5).

Large-scale randomized controlled studies of adjunctive clonazepam have not yet been done. While duration of benefit clinically appears to be prolonged, some reports suggest that symptom relief can be short lived. Not all schizophrenia with voices patients will benefit from adjunctive clonazepam. The controlled FDA approval studies of clonazepam for ordinary panic may promote optimism for schizophrenia and voices with panic, but not certainty. Despite the limited formal data, some preliminary usage guidelines have been proposed.[38]

Although clonazepam is a safe medication with proper dosing, supervision, and patient selection, there are a variety of concerns about its use.[39] The most common side effect is drowsiness after each dose increase. This tends to diminish or disappear after several days, but a small amount may linger. Because of this, patients and families should be warned, and caution exercised in the near term with alcohol, other sedating drugs, gait disorder, driving, power tools, and heavy equipment. There also appears to be long-term partial tolerance to the antianxiety effects, but not to the anti-panic effects (mediated by different GABA receptor subtypes). Caution is warranted with potentially noncompliant patients (consequent risk of withdrawal symptoms, especially at higher doses, and returning symptoms at any effective dose) and potentially violent patients (questions of disinhibition). Consideration is also needed for risks of drug diversion, and for medication loss due to theft in some patients.

Skilled psychotherapy is an essential part of treatment. In the earliest psychotic phases, a somewhat detached supportive psychotherapy helps establish a therapeutic alliance. With clinical improvement, therapy shifts to a more emotionally supportive, educational, and family model. Some patients will eventually benefit from more dynamic psychotherapy, with little risk of prompting clinical decompensation.

What Might Panic Psychosis Criteria Look Like?

Panic-like comorbidity with schizophrenia has been described since before panic disorder was named and officially recognized. For example, psychoanalyst Ping-Nie Pao wrote that, "When organismic panic prevails, all ego functions come to a standstill. As the ego loses its ability to discriminate internal imagery from external perception, the patient is hallucinating, whether or not he is able to communicate it verbally."[40] The further notion that panic might be a core component of some schizophrenia is also not new, but has not yet been specifically defined, well studied, or generally accepted. The concept is especially relevant, though, if it leads to more specific diagnosis and more effective treatment. And while there has been a small but steady flow of publications on both panic and schizophrenia and its treatment, the topics have been slow to gain research and clinical traction.

One way to start exploring a proposed definition of panic psychosis would be to start with existing DSM-5 criteria for schizophrenia, and then add additional criteria:

Proposed Panic Psychosis Criteria

1. DSM-5 inclusion and exclusion criteria for schizophrenia
2. DSM-5 criteria panic anxiety occurring during one or more of the following times:
   a. Concurrent with paroxysmal auditory hallucinations
   b. Concurrent with paroxysmal paranoid delusion exacerbations
   c. Pre-psychotic period
   d. Psychotic period
   e. Post-psychotic remission period
   f. Proven, accepted, and consented diagnostic panic challenge test
3. Either 2a or 2b or is clinically shown or suspected
   a. By focused, specific, and proven interview method
      i. During acute psychosis
      ii. During partial or full psychosis remission
   b. By accepted and proven biological test
      i. Unmedicated challenge test elicits concurrent panic with:
         1. Auditory hallucinations, and/or
         2. Paranoid delusions
      ii. Novel approach based on existing or future science
4. Panic psychosis can be comorbid with other psychiatric disorders:
   a. Obsessive-compulsive disorder
   b. Social anxiety disorder
   c. Melancholic depression
   d. Atypical depression
   e. Substance use psychoses
   f. Medical illness or medical treatment related psychoses

Summary

By itself, schizophrenia is a progressive and severely debilitating illness, and while panic anxiety is less severe, it nonetheless can cause significant distress and functional limitation. Not surprisingly, schizophrenia tends to be more severe when combined with comorbid panic anxiety. Panic diagnosis is difficult in psychotic patients, due to impaired cognition, fearfulness, insufficient attention by clinicians, and because panic can appear in psychotic form that masks the underlying panic.

Careful attention to panic diagnosis is highly beneficial to patients. When treated with fixed-dose q12h clonazepam (or some future replacement), many compliant patients with schizophrenia and voices can have substantial remission of positive and negative symptoms, as well as improvement in cognitive function. Combined with skilled psychotherapy, this approach can often allow return to a normal life.

Although clinical observation supports this approach, the research literature needs further publications, including randomized controlled studies. Meanwhile, further support is emerging from neurotransmitter and brain imaging research. With more sophisticated studies, there may be better futures ahead for many with schizophrenia.

References

1. American Psychiatric Association. *Diagnostic and Statistical Manual of Mental Disorders.* 5th ed. Arlington, VA: Author; 2013.
2. Tandon R, Nasrallah HA, Keshavan MS. Schizophrenia, "just the facts" 4. Clinical features and conceptualization. *Schizophr Res.* 2009;110(1–3):1–23. https://doi.org/10.1016/j.schres.2009.03.005.
3. Kahn JP, Meyers JR. Treatment of comorbid panic disorder and schizophrenia: evidence for a panic psychosis. *Psychiatr Ann.* 2000;30:29–33.
4. Tandon R, Keshavan MS, Nasrallah HA. Schizophrenia, "just the facts" what we know in 2008. 2. Epidemiology and etiology. *Schizophr Res.* 2008;102(1–3):1–18. https://doi.org/10.1016/j.schres.2008.04.011.
5. Anderson AE, Marder S, Reise SP, et al. Bifactor modeling of the positive and negative syndrome scale: generalized psychosis spans schizoaffective, bipolar, and schizophrenia diagnoses. *Schizophr Bull.* 2018;44(6):1204–1216. https://doi.org/10.1093/schbul/sbx163.
6. Quattrone D, Di Forti M, Gayer-Anderson C, et al. Transdiagnostic dimensions of psychopathology at first episode psychosis: findings from the multinational EU-GEI study. *Psychol Med.* 2019;49(8):1378–1391. https://doi.org/10.1017/S0033291718002131.
7. Kahn JP. *Angst: Origins of Anxiety and Depression.* New York: Oxford University Press; 2013.
8. Veras AB, Cougo S, Meira F, et al. Schizophrenia dissection by five anxiety and depressive subtype comorbidities: clinical implications and evolutionary perspective. *Psychiatry Res.* 2017;257:172–178. https://doi.org/10.1016/j.psychres.2017.07.048.
9. Kessler RC, Chiu WT, Jin R. The epidemiology of panic attacks, panic disorder, and agoraphobia in the National Comorbidity Survey Replication. *Arch Gen Psychiatry.* 2006;63(4):415–424. https://doi.org/10.1001/archpsyc.63.4.415.
10. Kahn JP. Sodikoff CL. Root Causes of Human Capital Effectiveness. 2006. Unpublished Data.
11. Kahn JP, Stevenson E, Topol P, et al. Agitated depression, alprazolam, and panic anxiety. *Am J Psychiatry.* 1986;143(9):1172–1173. https://doi.org/10.1176/ajp.143.9.1172.
12. Masdrakis VG, Legaki EM, Papageorgiou C, et al. Psychoticism in patients with panic disorder with or without comorbid agoraphobia. *Int J Psychiatry Clin Pract.* 2017;21(3):181–187. https://doi.org/10.1080/13651501.2017.1305111.
13. Goodwin RD, Fergusson DM, Horwood LJ. Panic attacks and psychoticism. *Am J Psychiatry.* 2004;161(1):88–92. https://doi.org/10.1176/appi.ajp.161.1.88.
14. Goodwin R, Davidson L. Panic attacks in psychosis. *Acta Psychiatr Scand.* 2002;105(1):14–19. https://doi.org/10.1034/j.1600-0447.2002.
15. Goodwin R, Lyons JS, McNally RJ. Panic attacks in schizophrenia. *Schizophr Res.* 2002;58(2–3):213–220. https://doi.org/10.1016/s0920-9964(01)00373-5.
16. Savitz AJ, Kahn TA, McGovern KE, et al. Carbon dioxide induction of panic anxiety in schizophrenia with auditory hallucinations. *Psychiatry Res.* 2011;189(1):38–42. https://doi.org/10.1016/j.psychres.2011.06.008.

17. Kahn JP, Bombassaro T, Veras AB. Comorbid schizophrenia and panic anxiety: panic psychosis revisited. *Psych Annals.* 2018;48(12):561–565.
18. Rapp EK, White-Ajmani ML, Antonius D, et al. Schizophrenia comorbid with panic disorder: evidence for distinct cognitive profiles. *Psychiatry Res.* 2012;197(3):206–211. https://doi.org/10.1016/j.psychres.2012.01.017.
19. Ongur D, Lin L, Cohen BM. Clinical characteristics influencing age at onset in psychotic disorders. *Compr Psychiatry.* 2009;50(1):13–19. https://doi.org/10.1016/j.comppsych.2008.06.002.
20. Ciapparelli A, Paggini R, Marazziti D, et al. Comorbidity with axis I anxiety disorders in remitted psychotic patients 1 year after hospitalization. *CNS Spectr.* 2007;12(12):913–919. https://doi.org/10.1017/s1092852900015704.
21. Ulas H, Alptekin K, Akdede BB, et al. Panic symptoms in schizophrenia: comorbidity and clinical correlates. *Psychiatry Clin Neurosci.* 2007;61(6):678–680. https://doi.org/10.1111/j.1440-1819.2007.01724.x.
22. Labbate LA, Young PC, Arana GW. Panic disorder in schizophrenia. *Can J Psychiatry.* 1999;44(5):488–490. https://doi.org/10.1177/070674379904400510.
23. Galynker I, Ieronimo C, Perez-Acquino A, et al. Panic attacks with psychotic features. *J Clin Psychiatry.* 1996;57(9):402–406.
24. Higuchi H, Kamata M, Yoshimoto M, et al. Panic attacks in patients with chronic schizophrenia: a complication of long-term neuroleptic treatment. *Psychiatry Clin Neurosci.* 1999;53(1):91–94. https://doi.org/10.1046/j.1440-1819.1999.00477.x.
25. Heun R, Maier W. Relation of schizophrenia and panic disorder: evidence from a controlled family study. *Am J Med Genet.* 1995;60(2):127–132. https://doi.org/10.1002/ajmg.1320600208.
26. Wolf DH, Satterthwaite TD, Loughead J, et al. Amygdala abnormalities in first-degree relatives of individuals with schizophrenia unmasked by benzodiazepine challenge. *Psychopharmacology (Berl).* 2011;218(3):503–512. https://doi.org/10.1007/s00213-011-2348-7.
27. Hodges LM, Fyer AJ, Weissman MM, et al. Evidence for linkage and association of GABRB3 and GABRA5 to panic disorder. *Neuropsychopharmacology.* 2014;39(10):2423–2431. https://doi.org/10.1038/npp.2014.92.
28. Long Z, Medlock C, Dzemidzic M, et al. Decreased GABA levels in anterior cingulate cortex/medial prefrontal cortex in panic disorder. *Prog Neuropsychopharmacol Biol Psychiatry.* 2013;44:131–135. https://doi.org/10.1016/j.pnpbp.2013.01.020.
29. Hasler G, Nugent AC, Carlson PJ, et al. Altered cerebral gamma-aminobutyric acid type A-benzodiazepine receptor binding in panic disorder determined by [11C]flumazenil positron emission tomography. *Arch Gen Psychiatry.* 2008;65(10):1166–1175. https://doi.org/10.1001/archpsyc.65.10.1166.
30. Xu MY, Wong AHC. GABAergic inhibitory neurons as therapeutic targets for cognitive impairment in schizophrenia. *Acta Pharmacol Sin.* 2018;39(5):733–753. https://doi.org/10.1038/aps.2017.172.
31. Chiu PW, Lui SSY, Hung KSY, et al. In vivo gamma-aminobutyric acid and glutamate levels in people with first-episode schizophrenia: a proton magnetic resonance spectroscopy study. *Schizophr Res.* 2018;193:295–303. https://doi.org/10.1016/j.schres.2017.07.021.
32. Seeley WW, Turetsky N, Reus VI, et al. Benzodiazepines in schizophrenia: prefrontal cortex atrophy predicts clinical response to alprazolam augmentation. *World J Biol Psychiatry.* 2002;3(4):221–224. https://doi.org/10.3109/15622970209150625.
33. Fatemi SH, Folsom TD, Thuras PD. $GABA_A$ and $GABA_B$ receptor dysregulation in superior frontal cortex of subjects with schizophrenia and bipolar disorder. *Synapse.* 2017;71(7). https://doi.org/10.1002/syn.21973.
34. Kahn JP, Puertollano MA, Schane MD, et al. Adjunctive alprazolam for schizophrenia with panic anxiety: clinical observation and pathogenetic implications. *Am J Psychiatry.* 1988;145(6):742–744. https://doi.org/10.1176/ajp.145.6.742.
35. Barbee JG, Mancuso DM, Freed CR, et al. Alprazolam as a neuroleptic adjunct in the emergency treatment of schizophrenia. *Am J Psychiatry.* 1992;149(4):506–510. https://doi.org/10.1176/ajp.149.4.506.
36. Nardi AE, Machado S, Almada LF, et al. Clonazepam for the treatment of panic disorder. *Curr Drug Targets.* 2013;14(3):353–364. https://doi.org/10.2174/1389450111314030007.
37. Pecknold JC. Survey of the adjuvant use of benzodiazepines for treating outpatients with schizophrenia. *J Psychiatry Neurosci.* 1993;18(2):82–84. Retrieved from https://www.ncbi.nlm.nih.gov/pubmed/8096393.

38. Szarmach J, Wlodarczyk A, Cubala WJ, et al. Benzodiazepines as adjunctive therapy in treatment refractory symptoms of schizophrenia. *Psychiatr Danub.* 2017;29(Suppl 3):349–352. https://www.ncbi.nlm.nih.gov/pubmed/28953789.
39. Quagliato LA, Freire RC, Nardi AE. Risks and benefits of medications for panic disorder: a comparison of SSRIs and benzodiazepines. *Expert Opin Drug Saf.* 2018;17(3):315–324. https://doi.org/10.1080/14740338.2018.1429403.
40. Pao PN. *Schizophrenic Disorders: Theory and Treatment from a Psychodynamic Point of View.* New York: International Universities Press; 1979.

CHAPTER 5

Persecutory Delusional Disorder and Social Anxiety

Thaysse Gomes Ricci ▦ Maria Rita Silva de Souza ▦ Aline França da Hora Amarães ▦ Kethlyn Carolina Motter ▦ André Barciela Veras

Abstract

Social anxiety disorder (SAD) is among the most frequent and consequential comorbidities in psychoses. It is vital to pay close attention to proper diagnosis and treatment. Persecutory Delusional Disorder (PDD) is often misdiagnosed as schizophrenia due to some overlapping symptoms, and despite the retention of more outwardly normal functioning in PDD. SAD is commonly characterized by increased concerns about the opinions of others, and any embarrassment or humiliation that could result. SAD often precedes Persecutory Delusional Disorder (PDD), a diagnosis where fears of hostile others become fixed false beliefs. This chapter focuses on information that points to a relationship between PDD and SAD, emphaszing the need for diagnosis, treatment, and the need for further research.

KEYWORDS

Social anxiety disorder	Persecutory delusional disorder	Comorbidity
Schizophrenia	Psychosis	

Persecutory Delusional Disorder

Delusional disorders are characterized by fixed beliefs based on bizarre interpretations of reality (despite evidence to the contrary), not related to daily life experiences, and not specific to a given cultural group. There are five major subtypes: erotomanic (i.e., an individual delusionally believes that another person is in love with them), grandiose (i.e., delusional belief of having exceptional talent, ideas, or important discoveries), jealous (i.e., delusional belief that their significant other is unfaithful), persecutory (delusional belief that he or she is being conspired against, cheated, spied on, followed, poisoned or drugged, maliciously maligned, harassed, or obstructed in the pursuit of long-term goals), and somatic (the delusion involves bodily functions or sensations), along with mixed type and unspecified type. In this chapter we will be focusing on persecutory delusional disorder (PDD), sometimes known as paranoid delusional disorder (see Table 5.1).

The PDD term was first formalized in DSM-III-R, after an extensive discussion on paranoia and its ill-defined use in common speech. Currently, PDD and paranoia are synonyms, and still stem from Emil Kraepelin's 1915 idea of paranoid disorder.

Persecutory DD is often misdiagnosed as schizophrenia due to some symptoms common to the two disorders.[1] This confusion resembles the historical notion that perhaps PDD is just a mild

TABLE 5.1 ■ **Diagnostic Criteria: Delusional Disorder**

DSM5 297.1 (ICD10 F22)

a. The presence of one (or more) delusions with a duration of 1 month or longer.
b. Criterion A for schizophrenia has never been met.
   Note: Hallucinations, if present, are not prominent and are related to the delusional theme (e.g., the sensation of being infested with insects associated with delusions of infestation).
c. Apart from the impact of the delusion(s) or its ramifications, functioning is not markedly impaired, and behavior is not obviously bizarre or odd.
d. If manic or major depressive episodes have occurred, these have been brief relative to the duration of the delusional periods.
e. The disturbance is not attributable to the physiologic effects of a substance or another medical condition and is not better explained by another mental disorder, such as body dysmorphic disorder or obsessive-compulsive disorder.

Persecutory type: This subtype applies when the central theme of the delusion involves the individual's belief that he or she is being conspired against, cheated, spied on, followed, poisoned or drugged, maliciously maligned, harassed, or obstructed in the pursuit of long-term goals.

Delusional Disorder (page 90—code 297.1, F22).
American Psychiatric Association. Schizophrenia spectrum and other psychotic disorders. In *Diagnostic and Statistical Manual of Mental Disorders*. 5th ed. 2013.https://doi.org/10.1176/appi.books.9780890425596.dsm02.

form of paranoid schizophrenia. Indeed, this outdated view was included in DSM-II.[2] Since then, rigorous research has shown that PDD and schizophrenia diverge in premorbid personality traits, marital status, hospitalization index,[3] and the fact that negative and cognitive symptoms are only pronounced in schizophrenia.[1]

An example of what seems to be continuing confusion nonetheless supports a higher level of cognitive symptoms in schizophrenia than in PDD. A factor analysis study compared schizophrenia subjects with and without comorbid social anxiety, but the latter group may actually have been inadvertently misdiagnosed PDD. If so, their data offers useful support for the clinically accepted distinctions between schizophrenia and PDD.[4]

The essential feature of PDD is the persistence of one or more delusions for 1 month or more without fulfilling any symptom from schizophrenia's criteria A. If there are hallucinations, they are not related to delusional themes, and they are of brief duration. Aside from the adverse consequences of delusions, other behavior and psychosocial abilities are not affected. This is in contrast to the functional decline of schizophrenia. Lastly, the symptoms must not be a consequence of substance use (see Chapter 8) or other mental or medical conditions (Chapter 9).

Certain duration and recurrence specifiers only apply after 1 year of illness, subdivided into acute (a period when the symptom criteria are fulfilled), partial remission (an improvement after a previous episode is maintained and full criteria are no longer met), and full remission (does not have any disorder-specific symptoms). These concepts characterize both first and multiple episodes, but continuous criteria fulfillment for most of the disease course is also possible.

Thinking epidemiologically, it is hard to know PDD's true population prevalence, in view of exclusion criteria, patient avoidance of treatment, and the common confusion with schizophrenia. PDD-like symptoms are common within other schizophrenia spectrum disorders, but those symptoms are different than a clear diagnosis of "pure" PDD. Nevertheless, DSM5 declares prevalence to be around 0.02%, while female-to-male ratio varies across studies between 1:18 and 3:1. The mean age of onset is 40 years and represents 1% to 4% of all psychiatric admissions. Importantly, it is difficult for people with PDD to seek treatment, as they remain substantially functional, yet cannot recognize the negative effects of their fears on relationships and employability. Basically, they cannot doubt their own fixed beliefs, and they strongly reject any opposing opinions. As a result, they commonly develop social isolation, depression, and even an exacerbation of prodromal social anxiety.

Social Anxiety Disorder

Social anxiety disorder (SAD), also known as "social phobia," is one specific kind of anxiety. SAD is characterized by great concern about others' opinions due to the fear of being embarrassed, diminished, harmed by someone, or humiliated. People with SAD are usually afraid of being embarrassed in social situations; therefore, they tend to avoid places or circumstances where they could experience painful anxiety episodes. For example, they may be very shy people who avoid meeting strangers, public speaking, and situations where they may feel evaluated by others. As a result, most people with SAD reduce their investment in social relationships, which can present problems for differential diagnosis of SAD and schizophrenia spectrum disorder.[5] Not surprisingly, people with SAD have smaller social networks than others.

For example, Hur et al.[6] demonstrated that individuals with higher levels of social anxiety spend significantly less time with close companions, and that this results from smaller social networks. Because of this, socially anxious subjects spend significantly less time with others, and derive less emotional benefit.[6]

According to DSM 5 (see Table 5.2), the essential feature of SAD is great fear or anxiety about social situations "in which the individual is exposed to possible scrutiny by others" (DSM 5,

---

TABLE 5.2 ■ **Diagnostic Criteria: Social Anxiety Disorder**

DSM-5 300.23 (ICD10 F40.10)

a. Marked fear or anxiety about one or more social situations in which the individual is exposed to possible scrutiny by others. Examples include social interactions (e.g., having a conversation, meeting unfamiliar people), being observed (e.g., eating or drinking), and performing in front of others (e.g., giving a speech).
   Note: In children, the anxiety must occur in peer settings and not just during interactions with adults.
b. The individual fears that he or she will act in a way or show anxiety symptoms that will be negatively evaluated (i.e., will be humiliating or embarrassing: will lead to rejection or offend others).
c. The social situations almost always provoke fear or anxiety.
   Note: In children, the fear or anxiety may be expressed by crying, tantrums, freezing, clinging, shrinking, or failing to speak in social situations.
d. The social situations are avoided or endured with intense fear or anxiety.
e. The fear or anxiety is out of proportion to the actual threat posed by the social situation and to the sociocultural context.
f. The fear, anxiety, or avoidance is persistent, typically lasting for 6 months or more.
g. The fear, anxiety, or avoidance causes clinically significant distress or impairment in social, occupational, or other important areas of functioning.
h. The fear, anxiety, or avoidance is not attributable to the physiologic effects of a substance (e.g., a drug of abuse, a medication) or another medical condition.
i. The fear, anxiety, or avoidance is not better explained by the symptoms of another mental disorder, such as panic disorder, body dysmorphic disorder, or autism spectrum disorder.
j. If another medical condition (e.g., Parkinson disease, obesity, disfigurement from bums or injury) is present, the fear, anxiety, or avoidance is clearly unrelated or is excessive.
Specify if:
Performance only: If the fear is restricted to speaking or performing in public.

Social Anxiety Disorder (page 90—code 297.1, F22).
American Psychiatric Association. Schizophrenia spectrum and other psychotic disorders. In *Diagnostic and Statistical Manual of Mental Disorders.* 5th ed. 2013. https://doi.org/10.1176/appi.books.9780890425596.dsm02.

2013, pg. 202). Examples include having a conversation, meeting new people, the feeling of being observed while drinking or eating, and performing in front of others.

The embarrassment is typically related to fear of being seen as somehow inferior. It can manifest in specific and varied places, including work, school, parties, and wherever public presentation is required. With an intense fear or anxiety of social situations, where the individual may be negatively evaluated by others, they may be afraid of being judged crazy, stupid, boring, or incapable, among others. The fear of embarrassingly negative evaluation can include fear that the anxiety itself will be noticed by others, not to mention such visible anxiety symptoms as blushing, sweating, switching words, and staring. Depending on the symptoms, people may avoid situations that could evoke those symptoms. An individual with trembling hands when anxious may avoid drinking, writing, or eating in public.[7]

PHENOMENOLOGY

Even when severe, SAD does not initially affect overall function. It occurs mainly with certain tasks, situations, and circumstances. Most of the time the socially anxious individual can realize that their fears and concerns are excessive and unreasonable, but when exposed to situations producing great anxiety, they can have a conscious perception that they are being judged by those around them.[5,8] This thought persists even if they ultimately decide that they are actually viewed quite positively. Successful entertainers with SAD are one such example.

Thus, it is not surprising that quasi-paranoid feelings can result from SAD fears. Since SAD patients often have self-referential ideas, they share certain cognitive processes with paranoid patients (PDD). To this point, Taylor and Stopa[9] suggest similarities in thoughts, behaviors, core beliefs, and assumptions in subjects with SAD and persecutory beliefs. Moreover, some SAD patients may become actually paranoid when they lose their conscious ability to moderate their social fears, and thus progress to a psychotic disorder.[5]

From an evolutionary perspective, SAD is associated with a fixed perception of inferiority (or inferior status) in the eyes of others. In consequence, some fear they may be pursued or humiliated by more powerful or confident individuals.[10] In the ancient past, social hierarchy kept everyone in line, and avoided too many cooks spoiling the broth. Community rank ensured that duties and obligations were accomplished with some degree of social harmony.

Other species also have social hierarchies, from the weakest to the strongest, inexperienced to experienced, and biologically shy to biologically confident. This ranking helps other species to reduce conflict, and thus better adapt as a group. More successful groups help to keep the species DNA alive.

On the other hand, we humans today are more conscious of our preferences, choices, and social rank aspirations. So, those with SAD in modern society may end up with an anxiety problem. When conflict between rational aspirations and biological instinct is resolved in favor of the aspirations, those with SAD may experience more anxiety than they expect, want, or can stand. This may lead to ongoing distress, or eventual limitation of their aspirations.[10]

With current technologies, we humans can try to overcome social anxiety and loneliness by increasing the number of linked friends, comments, or likes on social networks, as a representation of social acceptance, and thus of social rank. This is in addition to more long-standing stand-ins for rank such as the brand of your conveyance, your clothing and jewelry, where you live, and your occupation, all of which can be responsible for displaying (or "determining") your social status.

This is a mixed blessing for those humans with SAD: conscious reassurance of heightened social rank on the one hand, but increased risk of social anxiety and fear of embarrassment on the other. Ironically, some will have diminished social contact as a result. Individuals with SAD may worry about things that can go wrong, especially that they might be viewed as a social hierarchy impostor. An emotionally easier path is to "go unnoticed."[10] One study showed that people who are more easily and obviously embarrassed are considered more pleasant and trustworthy by others, which may reflect submissive and deferential behavior—and a self-perceived lower social ranking.[11]

DEMOGRAPHICS AND EPIDEMIOLOGY

SAD is a common mental disorder in the United States, with studies indicating a prevalence of 6.8% in 12 months.[12] In Asian countries, like Japan and Korea, the observed prevalence of SAD tends to be lower (0.2% to 0.6% in Korea, 0.8% in Japan). Yet from another perspective, 1% or more Japanese may suffer from tajin kyofusho (which approximates SAD) or hikikomori (severe social withdrawal that may include SAD). Meanwhile, Russia presents one of the highest levels (32.6%).[8]

Social anxiety is considered an early-onset disorder with a typically chronic course.[13] Some studies suggests that the most frequent age of onset is between 12 and 17 years old. Besides hereditary,[14] other factors, such as lower social class, poorer financial circumstances, limited education level, unemployment, and unmarried status, represent significant risk factors for the development of SAD. Also, SAD seems to be more prevalent in women than men; it is important to note that women tend to present themselves more frequently to health services than men, which may influence these results.[15]

Chronicity is supported by SAD studies that report a mean disease duration of more than 10 years.[16] Comorbidity with other mental disorders is common. The presence of comorbidities can range from 69% to 92% in cases of SAD, so that the presence of SAD alone would be somewhat uncommon.[15] A multinational population study suggested that approximately 50% of individuals with SAD also have other psychiatric diagnoses. Among them, the main associations were agoraphobia (21.6%), generalized anxiety disorder (13.5%), panic disorder (11.6%), and depression (10.2%).[17]

In addition, SAD is the second most common anxiety disorder (9.7%) in people with bipolar disorder.[18] Importantly, SAD commonly appears as a comorbidity in schizophrenia patients. In a study involving 207 patients with schizophrenia, 30 of them (14.5%) met criteria for SAD. SAD comorbidity is significantly correlated with the duration of untreated psychosis, intensity of psychiatric symptoms, poorer social functioning, and lower quality of life.[19]

Therefore, when comorbid with other disorders, SAD predicts poorer prognosis, increased chronicity and severity, and, in cases of depression, may increase the risk of suicide. SAD has a major negative social, educational, and occupational impact on the individual. It is associated with a higher prevalence of school dropout and greater risk of unemployment. This may result in significant community impact, since such patients often become dependent on others.[20]

Social Anxiety Disorder and Comorbidity in Schizophrenia

Aside from the frequent misdiagnosis of PDD as schizophrenia, SAD is one of the five most common comorbidities in schizophrenia. Deeper analysis is essential for understanding the interactions and co-occurrence of these two disorders. Research shows that SAD symptoms are very common in patients with schizophrenia, and 17% of the schizophrenia individuals are diagnosed with SAD.[21-23] Psychotic individuals manifest signs and symptoms of SAD much like individuals who only have SAD without comorbidity. Since psychotic symptoms are generally considered more significant and more clinically relevant, anxiety symptoms typically receive too little clinical attention.[23,24]

SAD in schizophrenia is associated with high suicide attempt risk, low quality of life, impaired social functioning, and low self-esteem, and is a major determinant of early schizophrenia.[25,26] In addition, comorbid SAD with schizophrenia may intensify the social stigmatization of psychotic individuals as useless or dangerous people. That type of experience can lead to avoidance of social situations and to distressing humiliation.[25,26] People with schizophrenia have diminished affection in relationships, just as those with SAD have diminished assertive behavior. Lysaker et al.[25,26] argues that the failure to recognize others' emotions makes social relationships difficult to navigate, so that interacting with others is a source of frustration, rather than a more satisfying relationship.

Several studies indicate that certain environmental factors may be related to the development of anxiety in schizophrenia. Exacerbated expression of emotions due to stressful and conflicting relationships between patients and their relatives results in more pronounced manifestations of anxiety and psychosis in patients diagnosed with schizophrenia,[27] as well as causing a significant increase in positive and psychotic symptoms.[28,29]

Not surprisingly, premorbid SAD influences schizophrenia onset and prognosis.[27,30] SAD also helps determine clinical presentation, such as greater anxiety and suspiciousness, increased concern about mind reading, and other ideas of reference.[3,31] With lesser self-esteem, increased self-referential paranoid concerns often focus on societal authority figures. Paranoid delusions in schizophrenia are typically related to fearful suspicion of malevolent observation by powerful authorities such as the CIA, FBI, religious figures, and aliens.[10]

Mild Quasi-Psychotic Features in Social Anxiety Disorder

Individuals with non-psychotic SAD may still have suggestive self-referential symptoms or ideas of reference. This may occur when SAD social fears overwhelm their mind's ability to consciously process those concerns. The greater an individual's ability to recognize that their concerns are internal exaggerations, the more these ideas are recognized as preoccupations or as anxiety. On the other hand, the lower their self-awareness, the greater the chance that their concerns seem real and immediate, resembling delusional self-referential experiences. These feelings of self-reference may be accompanied by more or less insight, varying across a broad range of perceived disapproval.

Veras et al.[32] discussed three possible explanations for psychotic manifestations in SAD patients. As noted above, the first is related to limited ability to evaluate internal anxious thoughts and feelings. The second possibility is that some stressors and intensifying factors could make individuals more likely to experience psychotic symptoms (as in PDD). Third and last, some patients may have SAD caused by a primary thought disorder abnormality leading to intense concern about others' opinions, with consequent psychotic self-reference rather than exaggerated anxiety.

The difficulty in distinguishing SAD from primary paranoia in some cases is related to the weakness of diagnostic constructs and current psychopathologic models, especially when the symptoms co-occur. In one sample of 161 patients, SAD patients had more cluster A personality disorders, especially paranoid personality.[33] Non-clinical samples have demonstrated that higher paranoid ideation is associated with higher levels of social anxiety, avoidance, apprehension, self-observation, and low self-esteem.[34]

Armando et al.[35] reported that the prevalence of psychotic-like experiences in individuals with SAD is indeed five times higher than controls. The same study reported that patients with SAD also had higher levels of depression, intolerance of uncertainty, and negative symptoms. Individuals with SAD and psychotic-like experience often have pessimistic thoughts and low self-esteem. When combined with deregulated affectivity, this plays an important role in paranoid delusions and psychotic symptoms.[36-38] These data are in accord with previous findings, which show that intolerance of uncertainty and related worries are linked to psychotic experiences, and that social anxiety increases the emotional responses to psychotic feelings.[39,40]

Social Anxiety Disorder and Persecutory Delusional Disorder: Chronology and Comorbidity

Even though SAD alone can be associated with increased quasi-paranoia, patients do tend to retain both societal function and awareness of the thoughts and emotions present in other people's minds (Theory of Mind).[10] True paranoid delusions with preserved cognition look very much like the DSM-5 criteria for "pure" PDD. Indeed, some patients with clinically diagnosed SAD much later develop DSM5 PDD.[5]

The median age that the first symptoms of SAD tend to appear is around 13 years old, and most have an age of onset between 12 and 17. Typically, SAD onset is preceded by earlier child-hood social inhibition or shyness.[7] The disorder may be influenced by humiliating or stressful situations, such as bullying, or embarrassment in front of other people. Moreover, since bullies tend to go after those who seem weak or shy, those with SAD are more likely to experience this kind of interpersonal trauma. Even a realistic hint of attack risk feeds into interpersonal fearful-ness, causing increased anxiety and self-referential paranoia.[41]

Onset in adulthood is relatively rare and more likely to occur after a highly stressful event or a major humiliation. Other risk factors for SAD development include temperamental behavioral inhibition, fear of negative evaluation, childhood maltreatment and adversity, and both genetic and physiologic traits. SAD and psychotic disorders share some common risk factors. Even with treatment, SAD tends to persist over time, although symptom severity can wax and wane, with some periods of significant exacerbation.

Observing the long-term course of diagnosed SAD patients, some of them later develop diag-nosed PDD.[5] From an evolutionary perspective, it is suggested that when conscious modulation of social ranking instincts linked to SAD are reduced by frontal cortex hypofrontality, then exaggerated amygdala reactivity of these patients may present as the actual delusions in PDD. This process may be further intensified by circumstances.[5] It is also possible that reduced conscious modulation of hypofrontality and adverse circumstances may be even more exacerbated if resulting anxiety feeds back to further "break up" self-consciousness, and lead to psychosis.[42] In the same report, researchers noted that some patients may develop moderate ongoing negative symptoms such as residual social withdrawal, apathy, and poor affective modulation. SAD, under certain conditions, may progress to PDD. Although further research is needed, PDD appears to be a psychotic form of SAD.[5]

Case Study Part I (Fictional Case)

Jonathan, a 37 year-old male, an online video game programmer, seeks psychiatric care at age 40 because of his mother's concern that he leaves their home only to buy essential food and supplies, although Jonathan does not believe that "this is a problem".

Jonathan's parents separated when he was 7 years old. His father was a harsh man who often quarreled with Jonathan's mother. His father often called him useless and claimed that no one liked him. A shy and quiet child, he was bullied at school. Older boys called him homophobic names and often mocked or pushed him. Over time, due to innate shyness as well as fears of bul-lying, he became socially isolated, often spending school recess alone, and with few friends.

During his adolescence he did not date because "just thinking about talking to girls" made his hands sweat and made him feel faint and very anxious. Every time he tried to talk to a girl he felt so anxious that he backed off, and eventually he stopped trying. A college degree in computer science taught him software coding skills. Right out of college, he found work in video game pro-gramming, which allowed him to work alone at home but with a bit of online socializing. Basically, he has mostly stayed inside his mother's house for about 15 years.

In his first interview he said that he prefers not to leave home because he has everything he needs there, and only leaves when he needs something. When he does go out, he has long felt non-paroxysmal tachycardia, anxiety, and excessive sweating. When he looks at people, he thinks they are saying something about him or making fun of him. He constantly thinks that he will embarrass himself in front of others, and thus be revealed as someone of little significance in society. He has no history of panic anxiety, even in social settings.

When reporting about his social world, he said that he usually communicates with his coworkers by text messaging, occasionally by telephone, and only infrequently by Skype when a video call is unavoidable. All of his work is done online from home. When he does need to deliver something for work, he uses a messenger service.

Jonathan had his first psychiatric contact at age 30. With a diagnosis of SAD, he complied with selective serotonin-uptake inhibitor (SSRI) antidepressant drug treatment for a few months, though he declined psychotherapy. He became a bit more social, outgoing, and cheerful, according to his mother. An online acquaintance even stopped by one day. Nonetheless, he quietly stopped medication, reporting later that he felt little real difference, and was concerned about what people would think about psychiatric medication use. When he leaves home now, he feels stressed out by the constant disrespect he suffers from men who walk past and look at him (sometimes looking at his back as he passes by). So, he sometimes leaves the shopping mall even before his shopping is completed. Early morning shopping trips can be easier, when there are fewer people around, and a bit easier still if he takes a shot of tequila beforehand.

Over time, SAD symptoms increased, and then psychotic symptoms began to appear. He started to think that people on the street could also read his mind, that television personalities were sending him special messages, and he was sure that the CIA was somehow behind it all—and they were waiting to pounce on any slight misstep. To protect himself, he reduced his already restricted activities. No more leaving the house: supplies were now ordered online and left at his doorstep. And to ensure no more Skype video sessions, he taped over the camera in his laptop. He also made sure to keep blinds drawn, and kept a baseball bat next to his bed. His mother's reassurances were met with an angry glare and even a fear that she was part of the problem. After years of concern, she was now quite alarmed.

How to Interview

Like any other psychiatric disorder, a well-detailed investigation of the individual's life history should include a primary focus on symptoms and their ages at onset. When thinking about SAD and PDD, it is important for the clinician to keep their symptoms and course clearly in mind.

The DSM-5 criteria present a clear summary of the core diagnostic features. In addition to these criteria, it is important to pay attention to additional important issues and aspects, as detailed below. As illustrated in the case, SAD and PDD are often associated with family and relational trauma history. To supplement the interview, there are scales that assess childhood trauma, for example the Early Trauma Inventory Self Report-Short Form.[43]

As our focus here is on the assessment of SAD with PDD, it is important to investigate early symptoms such as excessive shyness, fear of public speaking, limited social relationships, low self-esteem, fear that self-embarrassment will cause others to look down on them, and frequent concerns about critical observers.

On the other hand, when assessing the possibility of psychotic symptoms in patients with SAD, attention should be paid to the level of self-awareness, as this factor is important for discriminating true psychosis from overvalued fears. That distinction applies to exaggerated SAD symptoms, as well as the paranoid and self-referential fears of PDD. For example, can the patient offer or seriously consider alternative non-psychotic explanations?

Last but not least, PDD patients may have thoughts of violence, and sometimes act on them. Be sure to ask about violent and suicidal thoughts, how the patient can avoid violent behavior, and about access to weapons. Ask family members and friends about those same issues and any related history.

Importantly, psychotic patients require special interviewing skills and approaches. They may offer vague, evasive, confusing, and poorly detailed information, while being careful not to mention some of their most profound or fearful concerns. This makes interviewing difficult for basic issues, fears, comorbid symptoms, and even for earlier symptomatic history. Thus, in many cases, it is useful to revisit the full history after psychotic stabilization. In order to identify SAD symptoms in cooperative and open psychotic patients, scales can also be used, such as the Liebowitz Social Anxiety Scale (LSAS). This should be administered for both current symptoms and earlier pre-psychotic SAD symptoms.

Some basic guidelines for interviewing acutely psychotic patients are included near the end of Chapter 1.

Case Study Part II: Treatment

Due to the worsening of the patient's anxiety, irritability, and social withdrawal, the mother decided to make another try at treatment. In view of his heightened psychosis and baseball bat, he was admitted to an inpatient unit as a precaution. After an initial full clinical interview, treatment with aripiprazole was indicated in order to acutely diminish paranoia. Some initial softening of paranoia was noted within days. This took the form of less preoccupation, rather than less certainty. This partial improvement then allowed a more detailed interview, with additional information about symptom history and progression, as well as medical and personal history.

In view of his prior history of SAD (a chronic, and possible underlying, syndrome) fluoxetine 20 mg qd was also added, and expected to start helping about 4 weeks later. Since fluoxetine has a very long half-life, it is useful for patients at risk of noncompliance on discharge. And aripiprazole has the added benefit of enhancing SSRI treatment of SAD. At the same time, with an eye to possible future noncompliance, he was also started on injectable depot aripiprazole, requiring roughly monthly injections in the future.

In addition to drug treatment, psychotherapeutic follow-up based on either supportive dynamically informed technique or cognitive behavioral therapy is indicated in order to work on the recognition of dysfunctional symptoms and criticism regarding the condition and severity of the patient. Despite adhering to the treatment, Jonathan at first had difficulty attending psychotherapy sessions because he believed that people would know he was sick and make fun of him. As his condition improved, he began to appreciate the value of medication and therapy.

Over time, the subject showed increasing response to medication. Within a few months, his paranoid delusions remained, but were much less important to him. Meanwhile, his SAD had improved enough that he was more social than he had been in many years. Since he fully complied with treatment, these benefits remained for a long time. Ongoing psychotherapy helped him rebuild his life, drawing in part on his career success even during most of his illness.

Social Anxiety Disorder and Persecutory Delusional Disorder Treatment

It is common that people with SAD tend to shy away from treatment, and this is even more true for PDD. Usually, looking for a psychiatrist or psychologist initially increases anxiety, even if family is in charge. Medication treatment of SAD has shown great efficacy with the use of SSRI antidepressants, which work by increasing serotoninergic activity, but with anxiolytic effects only starting after 4 weeks. Benzodiazepines such as clonazepam may show modest initial benefit for anxiety, but they do little for core SAD concerns about embarrassment and avoidance, and have little role beyond initial treatment.

Psychotherapy associated with medication treatment has also been shown to be effective for SAD. The psychotherapeutic process helps the individual to understand and change patterns of shyness and avoidant behavior. Although the medications offer pharmacologic benefit, long-term psychotherapy should also be part of the treatment of individuals with SAD. Once you have a lifetime of experience with SAD, the beliefs become rooted in cognition as well as biology, but improve with time and thoughtfulness.

For PDD, treatment avoidance is far more pronounced. Special efforts are often required to engage the patient in treatment, and initial hospitalization is often the wise choice. Initial medication starts with an oral antipsychotic, and aripiprazole has advantages as noted above (fewer side effects, depot formulation available, enhancement of SSRIs for SAD). As appropriate (i.e., prior history of SAD, a chronic and possibly underlying syndrome), and with little downside risk, oral fluoxetine 20 mg can be added, with expectation of initial benefits 4 weeks later.

Reports have noted that patients diagnosed with schizophrenia and symptoms of SAD can be adjunctively treated with a SSRI. Choices of SSRIs include citalopram, escitalopram, fluoxetine, fluvoxamine, and sertraline.[44,45]

With these medications, delusions may start to become less important within a few days. Within months, delusions may fade to little importance, while SAD may continue to improve over the longer term. Psychotherapy is essential for compliance, making sense of illness history, and rebuilding a life.

Social Anxiety Disorder and Persecutory Delusional Disorder

While investigation of psychotic-like symptoms in SAD patients has been well reported in the literature, as well as studies of SAD concurrent with schizophrenia, there are few papers that address a progression of SAD to PDD. Patients with severe SAD symptoms often experience self-referential feelings. Such feelings may be accompanied by greater or lesser conscious assessment by the patient. Other works presented in this chapter point out that SAD and PDD are more than just consequences of stressful experiences: the disorders share common risk factors, and look like sometimes successive pathways of a common underlying psychopathologic process.

Although psychiatric diagnostic manuals long ago codified psychotic mood syndromes such as mania and delusional depression, companion psychotic anxiety disorders have been proposed but not yet accepted.[5] Limited controlled research is one reason, but PDD is considered rare, and such research has found little funding. Even so, limited research evidence as well as clinical observation strongly suggest that the SAD/PDD construct may improve treatment approaches. If warranted by further research, future DSM diagnoses might consider PDD as "psychotic social anxiety disorder." This codification seems to be in accordance with a dimensional diagnosis, reflecting the transition from SAD and PDD, and linking this anxiety disorder to the schizophrenia spectrum disorders.

Summary

SAD can be considered a lifetime disorder, in which the individual keeps himself trapped in his beliefs and fears, resulting in consequences for their personal, work, academic, and affective life. With the diagnostic description in the American Psychiatric Association's DSM-5, it is possible to document specific characteristics of SAD. However, additional symptoms may also occur with this disorder. Escalation to psychotic symptoms, as in PDD, can worsen symptoms, function, and prognosis. It seems more than plausible that recognition of this connection suggests a novel treatment approach worth careful evaluation. Further research is also needed to better evaluate, document, and detail the relationship between SAD and delusional disorder.

References

1. Marneros A, Pillman F, Wustmann T. Delusional disorders—are they simply paranoid schizophrenia? *Schizophr Bull.* 2010;38(3):561–568.
2. Kendler KS. The nosologic validity of paranoia (simple delusional disorder). A review. *Arch Gen Psychiatr.* 1980;37(6):699.
3. Hui CL, Lee EH, Chang WC, et al. Delusional disorder and schizophrenia: a comparison of the neurocognitive and clinical characteristics in first-episode patients. *Psychol Med.* 2015;45(14):3085–3095. https://doi.org/10.1017/S0033291715001051. Epub 2015 Jun 3 26036591.
4. Sutliff S, Roy MA, Achim AM. Social anxiety disorder in recent onset schizophrenia spectrum disorders: the relation with symptomatology, anxiety, and social rank. *Psychiatr Res.* 2015;227(1):39–45.
5. Veras AB, Souza TG, Ricci TG, et al. Paranoid delusional disorder follows social anxiety disorder in a long-term case series: evolutionary perspective. *J Nery Ment Dis.* 2015;203(6):477–479.
6. Hur J, DeYoung KA, Islam S, Anderson AS, Barstead MG, Shackman AJ. Social context and the real-world consequences of social anxiety. *Psychological Medicine.* 2019;1–12.
7. American Psychiatric Association. *Diagnostic and Statistical Manual of Mental Disorders.* 5th ed. Arlington, VA: Author; 2013.
8. Nardi AE, Quevedo J, Silva AG. *Transtorno de ansiedade social: teoria e clínica.* Porto Alegre: Artmed; 2014.
9. Taylor KN, Stopa L. The fear of others: a pilot study of social anxiety processes in paranoia. *Behav Cogn Psychother.* 2013;41(1):66–88.
10. Kahn JP. *Angst: Origins of Anxiety and Depression.* New York: Oxford University Press; 2013.
11. Feinberg M, Willer R, Keltner D. Flustered and faithful: embarrassment as a signal of prosociality. *J Pers Soc Psychol.* 2012;102(1):81–97.
12. Stein MB, Stein DJ. Social anxiety disorders. *Lancet.* 2008;371(9618):1115–1125.
13. Wittchen HU, Stein MB, Kessler RC. Social fears and social phobia in a community sample of adolescents and young adults: prevalence, risk factors and co-morbidity. *Psychiatr Danub.* 2009;21(4):520–524.
14. Chavira DA, Stein MB. Childhood social anxiety disorder: from understanding to treatment. *Child Adolesc Psychiatr Clin N Am.* 2005;21(4):520–524.
15. Fehm L, Pelissolo A, Furmark T, et al. Size and burden of social phobia in Europe. *Eur Neuropsychopharmacol.* 2005;15(4):453–462.
16. Wancara J, Fridl M, Friedrich E. Social phobia: epidemiology and health care. *Psychiatr Danub.* 2009;21(4):520–524.
17. Alonso J, Angermeyer MC, Bernert S, et al. 12 month comorbidity patterns and associated factor in Europe: results from the European Study of the Epidemiology of Mental Disorders (ESEMed) project. *Acta Psychiatr Scand Suppl.* 2004;420:28–37.
18. Pavlova B, Perlis RH, Mantere O, et al. Prevalence of current anxiety disorders in people with bipolar disorder during euthymia: a meta-analysis. *Psychol Med.* 2017;47(6):1107–1115.
19. Aikawa S, Kobayashi H, Nemoto T, et al. Social anxiety and risk factors in patients with schizophrenia: relationship with duration of untreated psychosis. *Psychiatr Res.* 2018;263:94–100.
20. Mochcovitch MD. Epidemiologia. In: Nardi AE, Quevedo J, Silva AG (orgs). *Transtorno de ansiedade social: teoria e clínica.* Porto Alegre: Artmed; 2014:23–27.
21. Cassano GB, Pini S, Saettoni M, et al. Multiple anxiety disorder comorbidity in patients with mood spectrum disorders with psychotic features. *Am J Psychiatr.* 1999;156(3):474–476.
22. Cosoff SJ, Hafner RJ. The prevalence of comorbid anxiety in schizophrenia, schizoaffective and bipolar disorder. *Austr N Z J Psychiarty.* 1998;32:67–72.
23. Dernovšek MZ, Šprah L. Comorbid anxiety in patients with psychosis. *Psychiatr Danub.* 2009;21(Suppl 1):43–50.
24. Braga RJ, Petrides G, Figueira I. Anxiety disorders in schizophrenia. *Compr Psychiatr.* 2004;45(6):460–468.
25. Lysaker PH, Yanos PT, Outcalt J, et al. Association of stigma, self- esteem, and symptoms with concurrent and prospective assessment of social anxiety in schizophrenia. *Clin Schizophr Relat Psychoses.* 2010;4(1):41–48.
26. Lysaker PH, Salvatore G, Grant ML, et al. Deficits in theory of mind and social anxiety as independent paths to paranoid features in schizophrenia. *Schizophr Res.* 2010;124(1–3):81–85.
27. Braga RJ, Reynolds GP, Siris SG. Anxiety comorbidity in schizophrenia. *Psychiatr Res.* 2013;210(1):1–7.
28. Glynn SM, Randolph ET, Eth S, et al. Patient psychopathology and expressed emotion in schizophrenia. *Brit J Psychiatr.* 1990;157:877–880.

29. Docherty NM, St Hilaire A, Aakre JM, et al. Anxiety interacts with expressed emotion criticism in the prediction of psychotic symptom exacerbation. *Schizophr Bull.* 2011;37:611–618.

30. Johnstone EC, Ebmeier KP, Miller P, et al. Predicting schizophrenia: findings from the Edinburgh high-risk study. *Brit J Psychiatr.* 2005;186:18–25.

31. Veras AB, Cougo S, Meira F, et al. Schizophrenia dissection by five anxiety and depressive subtype comorbidities: clinical implications and evolutionary perspective. *Psychiatr Res.* 2017;257:172–178. https://doi.org/10.1016/j.psychres.2017.07.048. Epub 2017 Jul 26 28763736.

32. Veras AB, Nascimento JS, Rodrigues RL, et al. Psychotic symptoms in social anxiety disorder patients: report of three cases. *Int Arch Med.* 2011;4:12.

33. O'Toole MS, Arendt M, Fentz HN, et al. Cluster a personality pathology in social anxiety disorder: a comparison with panic disorder. *Nord J Psychiatry.* 2014;68(7):460–463.

34. Martin JA, Penn DL. Social cognition and subclinical paranoid ideation. *Br J Clin Psychol.* 2001;40(Pt 3):261–265.

35. Armando M, Lin A, Girardi P, et al. Prevalence of psychotic-like experiences in young adults with social anxiety disorder and correlation with affective dysregulation. *J Nerv Ment Dis.* 2013;201(12):1053–1059.

36. Smeets F, Lataster T, Dominguez MG, et al. Evidence that onset of psychosis in the population reflects early hallucinatory experiences that through environmental risks and affective dysregulation become complicated by delusions. *Schizophr Bull.* 2012;38:531–542.

37. Thewissen V, Myin-Germeys I, Bentall R, et al. Instability in self-esteem and paranoia in a general population sample. *Soc Psychiatr Psychiatr Epidemiol.* 2007;42:1–5.

38. Wigman J, Lin A, Vollebergh W, et al. Subclinical psychosis and depression: co-occurring phenomena that do not predict each other over time. *Schizophr Res.* 2011;130:277–281.

39. Morrison AP, Wells A. Relationships between worry, psychotic experiences and emotional distress in patients with schizophrenia spectrum diagnoses and comparisons with anxious and non-patient groups. *Behav Res Ther.* 2007;45:1593–1600.

40. White R, Gumley A. Intolerance of uncertainty and distress associated with the experience of psychosis. *Psychol Psychother.* 2010;83:317–324.

41. Lopes BC. Differences between victims of bullying and nonvictims on levels of paranoid ideation and persecutory symptoms, the presence of aggressive traits, the display of social anxiety and the recall of childhood abuse experiences in a Portuguese mixed clinical sample. *Clin Psychol Psychother.* 2013;20:254–266.

42. Veras AB, Nardi AE, Kahn JP. Attachment and self-consciousness: a dynamic connection between schizophrenia and panic. *Med Hypotheses.* 2013;81(5):792–796.

43. Bremner JD, Vermetten E, Mazure CM. Development and preliminary psychometric properties of an instrument for the measurement of childhood trauma: the Early Trauma Inventory. *Depress Anxiety.* 2000;12:1–12.

44. Temmingh H, Stein DJ. Anxiety in Patients with Schizophrenia: Epidemiology and Management. *CNS Drugs.* 2015;29(10):819–832.

45. Roy MA, Demers MF, Achim AM. Social anxiety disorder in schizophrenia: a neglected, yet potentially important comorbidity. *J Psychiatr Neurosci.* 2018;43(4):287–288.

CHAPTER 6

Delusional Depression and Melancholia

Laiana A. Quagliato ▪ Rafael C. Freire ▪ Antonio E. Nardi

Abstract

Psychotic (delusional) depression may be a form of melancholia. Melancholia is characterized by a severe episode of sad or apprehensive, nonremissive, and nonreactive mood, with acute onset, for a period of at least 2 weeks and impairment of the individual's daily activities. In melancholia, there are still changes in the psychomotricity and vegetative symptoms, besides being able to attend with psychotic symptoms. Within the present diagnostic classification it is frequently seen in severely ill patients with major depression disorder. However, melancholia presents a distinctive biological homogeneity in clinical experience and laboratory test markers, and it is differentially responsive to specific treatment interventions. Hypercortisolemia (reflected in the dexamethasone suppression test), disturbances in sleep architecture, and other biological characteristics of melancholic patients should be further evaluated. Melancholia is a lifetime diagnosis, typically with recurrent episodes. Treatment of psychotic depression generally requires a combination of anti-psychotic and anti-depressant medications. Therefore, the adequate treatment and fast recognition of these conditions is imperative for a favorable outcome for the patient.

KEYWORDS

Major depressive disorder	Psychosis	Melancholia
Delusional depression	Diagnosis	

Psychotic (Delusional) Depression

The primary classification system for diagnostic classification in psychiatry is currently the *Diagnostic and Statistical Manual of Mental Disorders*, 5th edition (DSM5) of the American Psychiatric Association.[1] Although psychotic major depression is simply classified as a severe form of major depression in DSM5, psychotic major depression may represent a unique subtype of melancholic major depression with its own phenomenology, treatment response, and biology.[2] The course of major depression is predominantly chronic (although the melancholic subtype is typically acute), with considerable treatment resistance,[3] and depression is estimated to be the leading cause of disability in the year 2030.[4] Psychotic features occur in about 14% to 25% of patients with major depression.[5] Psychotic major depression may be associated with an especially chronic course, more frequent hospitalizations, higher risk of suicide, and greater disability than other forms of depression.[5]

In DSM5, psychotic symptoms, delusions, and hallucinations may be classified as congruent (delusions of guilt, ruin, nihilism, hypochondria, or derogatory or accusatory hallucinations) or incongruent with mood (persecutory delusions, self-referral, control, or hallucinations without affective content).[1] In psychotic depression, usually people have extraordinary delusions that they are worthless to society, guilty of horrifying crimes, undeserving of life, that their body is physically rotting away, and even that they are already dead (diagnosed as Cotard syndrome).[6]

The prevalence of depressive disorder with psychotic symptoms has been investigated in population studies. According to one US study, the prevalence of psychotic symptoms was about 14% among patients with major depression.[7] In a multicenter study conducted in Europe, the prevalence of psychotic symptoms in major depressive episodes was 18.5% and in the general population, 0.4%.[8] Another epidemiologic study in the UK found an incidence of psychotic depression similar to that of schizophrenia.[9] The presence of psychosis is greater in severe depressive episodes, but is also found in mild to moderate conditions.[8] Psychotic (delusional) depression is considered a severe form of melancholia.[6,10,11]

Melancholia

In DSM5, melancholia is only a specifier of major depressive disorder.[1] Melancholic depression, or depression with melancholic features, is a DSM5 subtype of clinical depression (Table 6.1). According to DSM5, melancholic features apply to an episode of depression that occurs as part of either major depressive disorder or bipolar disorder (Table 6.2).[1]

HISTORY OF THE DIAGNOSIS

The earliest medical records regarding melancholia date back to ancient Greece.[12] According to Hippocrates' theory of moods, the illnesses stemmed from changes in the moods that circulated in the human body, the "vital mood," and the melancholia (Melan = black, Cholis = bile), which was a consequence of excessive black bile in the brain.[12] This theory is an historical landmark of mankind, since from this point of view, disease ceases to have a supernatural connotation and starts to have a biological basis.[12]

Melancholia was seen as a quasipsychotic disorder, considered partial insanity, with delusions that were circumscribed rather than numerous and diverse.[13] The nihilism of melancholic depression is characterized by extreme pessimism and skepticism in the face of any possible situation or reality. Psychotic depression can include such bizarre nihilistic beliefs as being already dead (Cotard syndrome).

In 1899, Kraepelin amalgamated melancholic depressions and what would now be called bipolar depression into manic depressive illness.[14] Episodes of this new disorder were characterized by their acute onset and remission, ordinarily within a period of months.[14]

In the second decade of the 20th century, Schneider focused attention on the major psychopathologic features of melancholic states, such as lack of mood reactivity, diurnal variation of mood, and psychomotor retardation.[15] These were the hallmarks of what was termed "vital depression," in contrast to neurotic depression or depressive personality disorders.[15] Schneider's emphasis on clinical features laid the basis for the operational criteria that emerged in the 1980s in DSM.[16]

Melancholia presents a distinctive pattern of symptoms and signs. These include (i) mood state items (e.g., guilt, remorse and self-reproach, feelings of unworthiness and hopelessness, greater severity of depressed mood, non-reactivity of mood, loss of interest, anhedonia; distinctly gloomy quality, and greater suicidal ideation); (ii) vegetative items (e.g., loss of appetite and/or weight loss, insomnia, particularly terminal insomnia, diurnal variation with mood and/or energy

TABLE 6.1 ■ Diagnostic Criteria: Major Depressive Disorder

DSM5 296.2/296.3 (F32/F33)

A. Five (or more) of the following symptoms have been present during the same 2-week period and represent a change from previous functioning; at least one of the symptoms is either (1) depressed mood or (2) loss of interest or pleasure.
  1. Depressed mood most of the day, nearly every day, as indicated by either subjective report (e.g., feels sad, empty, hopeless) or observation made by others (e.g., appears tearful). (Note: In children and adolescents, can be irritable mood.)
  2. Markedly diminished interest or pleasure in all, or almost all, activities most of the day, nearly every day (as indicated by either subjective account or observation).
  3. Significant weight loss when not dieting or weight gain (e.g., a change of more than 5% of body weight in a month), or decrease or increase in appetite nearly every day.
  4. Insomnia or hypersomnia nearly every day.
  5. Psychomotor agitation or retardation nearly every day (observable by others, not merely subjective feelings of restlessness or being slowed down).
  6. Fatigue or loss of energy nearly every day.
  7. Feelings of worthlessness or excessive or inappropriate guilt (which may be delusional) nearly every day (not merely self-reproach or guilt about being sick).
  8. Diminished ability to think or concentrate, or indecisiveness, nearly every day (either by subjective account or as observed by others).
  9. Recurrent thoughts of death (not just fear of dying), recurrent suicidal ideation without a specific plan, or a suicide attempt or a specific plan for committing suicide.

B. The symptoms cause clinically significant distress or impairment in social, occupational, or other important areas of functioning.

C. The episode is not attributable to the physiologic effects of a substance or to another medical condition.

D. The occurrence of the major depressive episode is not better explained by schizoaffective disorder, schizophrenia, schizophreniform disorder, delusional disorder, or other specified and unspecified schizophrenia spectrum and other psychotic disorders.

E. There has never been a manic episode or a hypomanic episode.

American Psychiatric Association. Depressive disorders. In: *Diagnostic and Statistical Manual of Mental Disorders*. 5th ed. 2013. https://doi.org/10.1176/appi.books.9780890425596.dsm04.

TABLE 6.2 ■ DSM5 Specifiers for Depressive Disorders

Specify if:
With melancholic features:
A. One of the following is present during the most severe period of the current episode:
  1. Loss of pleasure in all, or almost all, activities.
  2. Lack of reactivity to usually pleasurable stimuli (does not feel much better, even temporarily, when something good happens).

B. Three (or more) of the following:
  1. A distinct quality of depressed mood characterized by profound despondency, despair, and/or moroseness or by so-called empty mood.
  2. Depression that is regularly worse in the morning.
  3. Early-morning awakening (i.e., at least 2 hours before usual awakening).
  4. Marked psychomotor agitation or retardation.
  5. Significant anorexia or weight loss.

American Psychiatric Association. Depressive disorders. In: *Diagnostic and Statistical Manual of Mental Disorders*. 5th ed. 2013. https://doi.org/10.1176/appi.books.9780890425596.dsm04.

worse in the morning); and (iii) certain other features (e.g., physical retardation, agitation, concentration difficulties, and psychotic features).[16] The core cognitions of melancholia include guilt ("burden"), loss of pleasure, and hopelessness.[6] These thoughts are amplified by melancholia and set the stage for a mindset that one's life will soon end.[6] Melancholia typically has an acute sudden onset, and a propensity to remit.[13] Although sometimes there is no apparent precipitant, it can be triggered by serious medical illness, or by other circumstances that suggest a sudden pointlessness to continued existence.

In 1980, although included as a specifier for depression in *Diagnostic and Statistical Manual of Mental Disorders*, 3rd edition (American Psychiatric Association), melancholia faded as a distinct diagnosis because its operational criteria overlapped heavily with those for major depressive disorder.[16] More recently, there has been a renewed interest in the diagnosis.[18]

The incidence of melancholic depression has been found to increase when the temperature and/or sunlight are low.[19] However, there is little research on lifetime prevalence of melancholic depression. One analysis, based on hospital first admissions for a historical cohort composed of 597 patients, found 83% had been diagnosed as having melancholia.[20] Of this sample, 20% had recurrent admissions for mood disorders, of which 31% were admitted for severe depression without psychosis and 69% were admitted for depressive psychoses.[20] There were no admissions for mild or moderate depressive disorders.[20] A 2008 analysis of a large study of patients with unipolar major depression found a rate of 23.5% for melancholic features.[21]

The disorder can start with no obvious precipitant; almost half of patients had an illness episode lasting less than 6 months, and two-thirds had recovered within a year.[20] Melancholia is more common in the elderly, and incidence is higher in women. However, it is especially common in recently retired men.[6] People with prior psychotic symptoms may also be more susceptible to this disorder.[22]

MELANCHOLIA, DEPRESSION, AND PSYCHOSIS

Several psychiatrists contributed to better characterize melancholic and depressive disorders. In 1907, Kraepelin provided a simple division of "depressive states" with an emphasis on psychomotor change, describing those with "simple retardation unaccompanied by any hallucinations or delusions" and a "delusional form," characterized by the "presence of varied depreciatory delusions, especially of self-accusation and of a hypochondriacal nature, in addition to the evidence of retardation."[14] The British psychiatrist Maudsley similarly subtyped "melancholia" and "melancholy with delusions" (Table 6.3).[23]

The development of delusions in the context of a depressive episode as well as the emergence of depressive symptoms during a psychotic episode are both common. In fact, previous analyses conducted in large samples have considered mood symptoms as one of the dimensions of schizophrenia, alongside positive and negative symptoms.[24] Depressive symptoms

---

TABLE 6.3 ■ **DSM5 Specifiers for Depressive Disorders**

Specify if:
With psychotic features: Delusions and/or hallucinations are present.
With mood-congruent psychotic features: The content of all delusions and hallucinations is consistent with the typical depressive themes of personal inadequacy, guilt, disease, death, nihilism, or deserved punishment.
With mood-incongruent psychotic features: The content of the delusions or hallucinations does not involve typical depressive themes of personal inadequacy, guilt, disease, death, nihilism, or deserved punishment, or the content is a mixture of mood-incongruent and mood-congruent themes.

American Psychiatric Association. Depressive disorders. In: *Diagnostic and Statistical Manual of Mental Disorders*. 5th ed. 2013. https://doi.org/10.1176/appi.books.9780890425596.dsm04

occur in all stages of that disease, especially in the prodromal period, and during the psychotic episode.[24] Depressive symptoms also occur in stable patients, and the occurrence rates are well above the normal population.[24] The frequency of depressive episodes in stable schizophrenic patients is quite high, ranging from 16.5% in cross-sectional studies to 65% in 3-year follow-up studies.[24]

Longitudinal studies of schizophrenia have considered concurrent depression as an indicator of unfavorable prognosis, associating it with reduced response to medications, impaired social performance, higher rates of relapse, and longer hospitalizations.[24,25] Depression has been associated with poorer quality of life, impairment of cognitive functions, and suicide.[24,25] Approximately 10% of patients with schizophrenia commit suicide, and in more than 60% of these patients, suicide is associated with depressive symptoms.[24] Patients with depressive and psychotic symptoms often present an emotionless exterior but with pronounced internal delusions, reminiscent of masked delusional depression.[27]

Melancholia: Secondary Signs and Symptoms

Melancholia is characterized by a severe episode of sad or apprehensive, nonremessive, and nonreactive mood, with acute onset, for a period of at least 2 weeks and impairment of the individual's daily activities.[28] Melancholia also includes changes in psychomotor activity and vegetative symptoms, besides the possibility of psychotic symptoms.[28] The main characteristics that separate melancholic depression from non-melancholic depression are psychomotor retardation, pervasive sad mood, lack of reactivity, and lack of interest.[28] Psychomotor retardation and delusional symptoms are cardinal symptoms in this distinction.[28]

Other clinical differences are also described; those with melancholia are more likely to report such clinical features as anhedonia and anergy than those with lesser depressions. The condition is associated with a seemingly lower importance of stressful life events, lower rates of personality disorders, lower family history of alcoholism, and higher rates of suicide when compared with non-melancholic depression.[10,29] Likewise, there is evidence for differential response to treatment: there are many studies suggesting a diminished response of melancholia to psychotherapy, and a superior response to antidepressant medication.[30]

Even with somewhat varying clinical definitions, melancholic depression has been held to differ from non-melancholic depression across a number of biological parameters. These differences include (a) genetic: with an association of the melancholic subtype and the long allele of the serotonin transporter gene[31]; (b) biochemical: altered signal transduction in fibroblasts[32]; (c) anatomic: reduction of hippocampal volume[33]; (d) endocrine: an increased rate of dexamethasone nonsuppression[34]; and (e) circadian rhythm: as measured by polysomnography.[35]

Melancholia and Psychosis: A Continuum?

Mehl et al.[36] reported that persecutory delusions were independently predicted by personalizing bias for negative events and by depression in 258 patients diagnosed with schizophrenia. Some investigations indicate that persecutory delusions are associated with abnormal attention to threat-related stimuli: an explanatory bias toward attributing negative outcomes to external causes and biases in information processing relating to self-concept.[37] It is hypothesized that in delusional patients, activation of self-discrepancies by threat-related information triggers defensive explanatory biases, which have the function of reducing the self-blame, but lead instead to persecutory ideation.[37] Symptoms such as purposelessness are common in melancholia and delusional depression, and might be related to diminished coping and psychotic experience. The delusions and hallucinations may both cause or reflect greater psychological distress, such as the obsessional guilt and perceived victimization common to delusional depression.[2,38]

Mild Psychosis-like Features in "Nonpsychotic" Cases

A comprehensive list of clinical features confirmed that "nonpsychotic" melancholia cases evidenced greater psychomotor change, and while they reported a more severe mood disturbance, it was distinguished more by sustained duration than by severity.[27] However, they were no more likely to report greater numbers of vegetative features (e.g., appetite or weight change, insomnia). Additionally, both constipation and an absence of diurnal variation in mood were more likely to be reported by nonpsychotic subjects.[27]

Prepsychotic Onset Comorbidity

Melancholia is an acute syndrome.[39] However, in a significant number of cases we find a certain general type of personality and habits of life. A review of the patient's previous personality and temperament often show that he/she has been an inhibited type of individual with a tendency to seriousness, rigidity, humorlessness, and over-conscientiousness.[40,41] Daily life habits have been narrowly focused, somewhat stereotyped, and devoid of diversions. Frequently he/she has been a loyal subordinate, meticulous with details, rather than an aggressive leader.[41] The narrow range of interests, modest adjustment skills, asocial trends, inability to maintain friendships, intolerance, and sometimes middling adult sexual adjustment are frequent personality concomitants.[41,42] Likewise, there may be a rigid ethical code, proclivity for saving, profound reserve, significant sensitivity, outward evidence of anxiety, over-conscientiousness, and the meticulousness about relationships and work.[41]

Fictional Case History

IDENTIFICATION: Anne, 62 years old, female, white, owner and headmaster of a private school.

CHIEF COMPLAINT: "I do not want to live anymore."

HISTORY OF THE CURRENT ILLNESS: Anne attended the psychiatric consultation reporting that she had been feeling discouraged, tearful, sad, and "angry with the people around her" for the past 6 months. It began about when her husband of 40 years died suddenly after years of progressive cardiac failure. Anne then had trouble keeping up with her work: "Doctor, I cannot do anything I did before. My life is misery, I am a worthless waste of biology." The early and terminal insomnia as well as anorexia and progressive weight loss became a constant in her life. However, what others noted most was her newfound social isolation. Anne does not want to continue living, feels wronged by God, and thinks she is alone because of unhelpful coworkers and family.

As time passed, Anne became increasingly dysfunctional, restless, exhausted, and brooding. What sleep she had was easily disturbed and not at all refreshing. Anne forced herself to get out of bed, couldn't concentrate, struggled to remember things, couldn't make decisions, and became convinced of rapidly progressive dementia. Even though her staff saw that she was still able to effectively run the school despite her condition, she was convinced that her contribution was nonexistent, and the school, staff, and students would be better off without her.

Upon psychiatric examination, Anne is severely inhibited psychomotorically, physically rigid, and without affective responsiveness. As she tries to cooperate, her facial expression is frozen, and there are long pauses as she tries to answer questions. She reports that she has lost the ability to rejoice or cry. Her most important themes include her fears of failing her school, overburdening her son, and altogether failing at her own purpose and existence. As fear of financial ruin becomes overwhelming, thoughts of a hopeless future turn into a fixed delusion of impending financial ruin, despite her financial assets. Finally, Anne is convinced that her inner organs are rotting away, and that the certainty of her imminent death would be a relief to everyone. She had no prior history of mania or other psychiatric diagnosis or treatment.

PERSONAL HISTORY: Born in Rio de Janeiro, Anne is the eldest of five children. Childhood psychomotor and cognitive development was within the normal range. She was raised only by her mother, and had no contact with her father. During her childhood she always felt alone, since "her brothers did not pay much attention to her." Anne commented that as a shy child, she had few friends during childhood and adolescence, and limited social relationships with other relatives. Despite a strong education, she did not easily assimilate new ideas or adapt to new environments. Throughout her life, she was fastidious but conservative about personal appearance, and meticulous about the orderliness in her quarters. She presented personal thoughts from a pessimistic perspective, and considered herself a "perfectionist." Anne had no stable romance until age 24, when she met Nathan, whom she married and with whom she had a son. Her husband was her pillar of strength. After his death, Anne continued to live in the same apartment. With her son working in Germany, she currently lives alone. In the midst of her overwhelming loss, she has few social resources to draw upon.

The Psychiatric Interview and Assessment

A main objective of the psychiatric interview is to establish the diagnostic hypothesis. This requires a thorough psychiatric evaluation and differential diagnosis, including comorbidities. For severe depression or first-episode psychosis, interview data must include current illness and prior illness signs and symptoms (including bipolar mania), disease onset, severity, and evolution. Information about personal history should include pre-morbid functioning, life events, stressors, and medical illnesses that might be related to the present illness.

This initial assessment should be viewed as a process for precise syndromal diagnosis, with attention to potentially causal medical conditions, including neurologic disorders and psychoactive substances use. The psychiatrist, when facing a first psychotic episode, must always investigate the possibility of a general medical condition, especially when patient or family report occurrence of physical signs and symptoms during or immediately prior to psychiatric manifestations, atypical psychiatric manifestations, later age at onset, or poor response to initial treatment.[43]

At the same time, keep in mind that true melancholic and delusional depressions are often triggered by serious medical illness. In DSM5, unipolar major depression with psychotic features is a severe subtype of unipolar major depression. Psychotic symptoms of delusions and/or hallucinations are usually consistent with depressive themes of guilt, worthlessness, and ruin.

Besides clinical history and medical review of systems, laboratory tests are useful for detecting some medical conditions. Commonly used tests examine: complete blood count; fasting glycemic level; electrolytes; autoimmune diseases; HIV and syphilis serology; and kidney, liver, and thyroid function. Computed tomography or magnetic resonance imaging help to detect brain injury, and are especially important in the presence of neurologic signs and symptoms, atypical presentations of psychosis, symptoms suggestive of delirium, and in patients over 50 years of age.[44] All abnormalities should be followed up in concert with appropriate medical specialists, but do not automatically preclude psychiatric diagnosis.

Some basic guidelines for interviewing acutely psychotic patients are included near the end of Chapter 1.

The Melancholic Patient's Interview

On interview, a severely depressed patient may have impaired concentration, anergia, diminished motivation, and psychotic preoccupation, and thus provide very little information. Since the interview will often be shorter than usual, it may be best to avoid too many open-ended questions and focus instead on specific and direct questions. Interventions that reflect empathy for patients' perceived despair, hopelessness, low self-esteem, and future prospects may improve the quality of the interview data. For suicide risk assessment, it is essential to pose direct questions about ideation, plans, and previous attempts in this high-risk group. However, since the most suicidal patients may offer no direct confirmation of their thoughts and plans, it is also essential to listen for risk with a third ear. Similarly, many will hesitate to disclose delusions and hallucinations.

If some topics cause patient discomfort, a brief detour to more neutral topics may help. As a rule, start with more positive topics, then move to neutral areas, and finally to those that are more emotionally charged. In looking for positive aspects of the patient's current perspective, you can say: "Tell me what you appreciate about yourself." When feelings or cognitions require clarification or elaboration, you can say: "What did you feel at that moment?" or "What went through your mind?"

If patients hint at delusional themes during the initial interview, this presents an opportunity to return to that theme later for elaboration. Eventually, the interview should explicitly ask about possible delusional concerns. Those concerns generally reflect a severely pessimistic view of life, guilt, health, financial status, and related human concerns and fears. The delusional nature of those thoughts is determined by the degree of conviction, uncorrectability, dismissal of contrary evidence, and any resulting relevance for action or resolute passivity.[45] As melancholic and delusional thoughts drive away hope, the future becomes increasingly hopeless and frightening.[45,46] The delusional fear of suffering from an incurable physical disease is supported by perceived physical heaviness and lassitude, vegetative changes, out-of-body experiences, and depersonalization.[45,46] Patients can experience these internal physical symptoms as proof of hopeless illness, and will sometimes even convince family and other physicians that they can never recover.[45,46]

Patients who are primarily focused on their interpersonal relationships and responsibilities are increasingly concerned about their depressive inhibition and concerns about their failure to fulfill their personal obligations.[45,46] Fears of failing, burdening, or hurting a spouse, children, or family or of having harmed them in the past lead to delusions of guilt. For the religious faithful, failure begets delusions of sin before God.[45,46] These processes can lead to nihilistic preoccupation with suicide.[45,46]

Moments of temporary silence during the interview may evoke some patient anxiety, but also allow reflection and thus greater openness about topics under discussion. Silences may also reflect patient apprehension about a difficult issue—due to guilt, fear, mistrust, deliberate omission, or simply resistance.

Prolonged silences should be avoided, as they can lead to a break in interview communication and patient (or physician) resentment. Without waiting too long, say: "I realize that it is difficult to speak…" It is also important to remember that patients with severe depression may be stuporous, or even mute. In these cases, silence may represent a symptom of the psychopathologic picture that the patient presents.

Tools to Screen for Psychotic Depressive Patients

Some tools are available to help screen for psychotic depression. For instance, the Psychotic Depression Assessment Scale (PDAS), the Brief Psychiatric Rating (BPRS-5) subscale of the PDAS, and the Calgary Depression Scale for Schizophrenia (CDSS) may be used to assess psychotic depression.[47,48] Specifically designed for individuals with schizophrenia, the Calgary Depression Rating Scale was originally developed to address the issue of the overlap between depression and negative symptoms and has become the recommended scale to assess the severity of depression in schizophrenia.[47]

Results of these assessments might be biased by patient feelings of despair, hopelessness, low self-esteem, and pessimism about themselves, the world around them, and their future. In addition, patients with psychotic depression may have profound cognitive impairment. For example, one study showed that delusional depression is accompanied by deficits in visual memory, visuo-constructive abilities, speed of cognitive processing, and executive functions—all of which could make screening tools problematic.[49] Furthermore, delusional depressive patients might have increased mistrust, leading to evasive answers and avoidance of eye contact.

Case Report Part II: Treatment

With diagnosis of a currently severe depressive episode with psychotic symptoms, Anne begins medication treatment with lorazepam 0.5 mg two times a day as a fixed-dose anxiety medication and Zopiclon 7.5 mg as a sleeping pill. Most importantly, perphenazine 8 mg four times a day is used as an antipsychotic, and amitriptyline 150 mg daily is used as an antidepressant.

Benzodiazepines offer some initial reduction of pessimism, as well as improved sleep duration. Anne's son, in family counseling, confirms that Anne's business is organized and financially sound. Psychomotor inhibition slowly improves over the course of treatment. Perphenazine starts a gradual reduction in delusions, and they eventually fade to unimportance. When the amitriptyline starts to work in the fourth week of treatment, sleep duration, appetite, and psychomotor function return to normal. Depressed mood gradually fades away, and some joy later returns. Lorazepam is reduced and later discontinued. Anne retains slight residual symptoms in the form of increased irritability, exhaustibility, and reduced resilience. She will continue treatment in an outpatient clinic during her further recovery.

TREATMENT

Delusional depressive and melancholic patients respond better to broad-action tricyclic antidepressants than to narrow-action antidepressants, for instance serotonin reuptake inhibitors.[50] In comparison to those with non-melancholic mood disorders, melancholic patients rarely respond to placebos, psychotherapies, or social interventions alone.[30] Some authors advocate electroconvulsive therapy as a rapid treatment for melancholia; this can also be considered a first-line treatment for delusional depression,[51] along with subsequent medication.

In mixed-aged samples, combination treatment using a heterocyclic antidepressant or selective serotonin-reuptake inhibitor and perphenazine at doses of 32 mg/day or greater is associated with response rates exceeding 50%.[52] However, 40% of subjects who receive combination therapy with a conventional antipsychotic medication developed mild-to-moderate tremor or rigidity during a 5-week trial.[52]

Melancholia is a lifetime diagnosis because of frequent recurrent episodes.[53] Adequate treatment and fast recognition of this condition are imperative for favorable outcomes. For patients with severe, psychotic, or repeated episodes, ongoing antidepressant prophylaxis is advised.[54]

Suicide Risk Assessment

Patients with melancholia have an increased risk of suicide compared to the general population.[55] Investigations demonstrated that patients with depression with melancholic features had a greater prevalence of suicidal ideation.[55,56] Furthermore, patients with delusional depression are at a twofold higher risk, both during their lifetime and in the acute phase, of committing a suicidal attempt than patients with non-delusional depression.[55] There were no differences in suicidal tendencies between mood-congruent and mood-incongruent psychotic depressive patients. Delusional depression patients have a significantly higher level of violent suicide attempts.[57] Furthermore, patients with delusional depression committed more severe suicidal attempts when compared with non-delusional depressive patients.[58] Similarly, psychological autopsy of completed suicides found that psychotically depressive patients more frequently used violent methods than their non-psychotically ill counterparts.[59]

It is not clear why the presence of psychotic features should be associated with this increased sui-cidal risk in delusional depressive patients.[55,60] Many factors have been suggested. The association of psychosis with depression is often associated with an overall greater depression severity, which might contribute to higher levels of suicide attempts.[55] However, there are also reports that when delusional depressive and non-delusional depressive patients suffered from depressive episodes of equal severity, the delusional depressive group still had higher levels of suicide attempts.[61] Most likely, then, this elevated risk might more likely be due to psychosis per se (e.g., command hallucinations, delu-sional ideas), pronounced guilt feelings, impulsivity, or greater executive dysfunction (closely linked with psychosis), which interferes with rational problem-solving abilities.[55] Additionally, delusional depression's higher levels of psychomotor disturbance (i.e., agitation) and longer duration of depres-sive symptoms might play a role in increasing the rate of suicide attempts.[55] Detailed and thoughtful suicide risk assessment is imperative with melancholic or delusional depression patients, along with effective treatment and suicide risk management plans.[26] Even when no suicide risk is elicited, hos-pitalization should still be carefully considered for delusional depression.

Diagnostic Syndrome

Delusional depression is commonly regarded as a psychotic form of melancholic depression, despite DSM5's inclination to lump many forms of depression together as major depression. Importantly, melancholia presents a distinctive biological homogeneity in clinical experience and laboratory markers and is differentially responsive to specific treatment interventions. Melancholia has characteristic clinical features, including:

1. Psychomotor disturbance expressed as retardation or as spontaneous agitation.
2. Disturbances in affect disproportionate to stressors, marked by blunted emotional response, and nonreactive mood.
3. Reduced concentration.
4. Vegetative dysfunction manifested as interrupted sleep, loss of appetite and weight, reduced libido, and complaints about low energy, especially in the morning.
5. Although psychosis is not necessarily a feature of melancholia, it is often present. Nihilistic convictions of hopelessness, guilt, sin, ruin, or disease are common psychotic themes.

Several biological markers are frequently found in melancholic patients compared to other forms of depressive illness:

1. Hypercortisolemia is common in melancholia and relatively uncommon in non-melancholic mood disorders. The hypercortisolemia is demonstrated in the dexametha-sone suppression test.[62] Hypercortisolemia and its failure to be suppressed by exogenous steroid administration is characteristic of patients with melancholia, and studies have dem-onstrated that this abnormality is normalized with effective electroconvulsive therapy.[63] Interestingly, similar cortisol abnormalities seem to cause death in spawning salmon, and in two species of newly mated male marsupial mice.[6] A return of the abnormality after treatment cessation heralds relapse of the disorder.[63] However, clinical use of the DST for melancholia faded when studies of DSM-III[17] major depression found little value for that more broadly defined diagnosis.[63]
2. Psychomotor disturbances can include physical retardation, including immobility, slumped posture, slower movement, and muteness.[64]
3. Characteristic disturbances in sleep architecture, with reduced rapid eye movement (REM) latency, increased REM time, and reduced deep sleep.[65]
4. Markers of inflammation implicated in depression were quantified as higher in melan-cholic patients compared to non-melancholic patients.[66] In pursuing an autoimmune

contribution, melancholic patients were more likely to test positive for a 5-hydroxy-tryptophan antibody compared to non-melancholic and control participants.[67,68]

5. Low plasma serotonin level predisposes to melancholia.[69]

6. Neuroanatomically, melancholic patients had less gray matter volume in the left posterior insula and more white matter volume in the upper brainstem tegmentum compared to controls,[70] less overall gray matter volume compared to controls,[70] and evidenced more EEG abnormalities during consummatory reward tasks.[71,72]

7. Clinical genetic studies suggest a familial aggregation and a considerable heritability of psychotic depression partly shared with schizoaffective disorder, schizophrenia, and affective disorders.[73–75] Molecular genetic studies point to potential risk loci of psychotic depression shared with schizoaffective disorder, depression, bipolar disorder, and schizophrenia (6p, 8p22, 10p13-12, 10p14, 13q13-14, 13q32, 18p, 22q11-13) and several vulnerability genes possibly contributing to an increased risk of psychotic symptoms in depression (e.g., *BDNF, DBH, DTNBP1, DRD2, DRD4, GSK-3beta, MAO-A*).[73,76,77] The *5-HTT, DTNBP1,* and *TPH1* gene variation are implicated in pharmacogenetic investigations, and in the mediation of antidepressant treatment response in psychotic depression.[73,78] Genetic factors are suggested to contribute to the disease risk of psychotic depression in partial overlap with disorders along the affective-psychotic spectrum.[73,78] The transition from nonpsychotic depressive disorder to a psychotic form is more likely to occur in patients with genetic markers for frontal cortex hypofrontality or increased dopaminergic activity.[6,38]

Future research should be performed in order to identify specific melancholia characteristics. Increased research on this serious and debilitating disorder is important, so that melancholia be better recognized as a distinct, identifiable, and specifically treatable affective syndrome.

Summary

Melancholia is a lifetime diagnosis, typically with recurrent episodes. Within the present classification it is frequently seen in severely ill patients with major depression and with bipolar disorder. Therefore, a detailed interview assessing suicide risk and presence of delusions and hallucinations is important to help the physician in melancholia's diagnostic and in the patient's treatment. Hypercortisolemia (reflected in the dexamethasone suppression test), disturbances in sleep architecture, and other biological characteristics of melancholic patients should be further evaluated. Therefore it is important that future diagnostic manuals classify melancholia and delusional depression as distinct, identifiable, and treatable affective syndromes, rather than as just specifiers within major depression. This would reduce the odds that these conditions will be underdiagnosed and underreported by physicians, and allow improved treatment for these debilitating disorders.

References

1. American Psychiatric Association. *Diagnostic and Statistical Manual of Mental Disorders (DSM5®)*. American Psychiatric Pub; 2013, ISBN:0890425574.

2. Rothschild AJ. Challenges in the treatment of major depressive disorder with psychotic features. *Schizophr Bull.* Jul 2013;39(4):787–796. (Print)0586-7614.

3. Fava GA, Ruini C, Belaise C. The concept of recovery in major depression. *Psychol Med.* 2007;37(3):307–317. (Print)0033-2917.

4. Lépine JP, Briley M. The increasing burden of depression. *Neuropsychiatr Dis Treat.* 2011;7(Suppl 1):3–7. (Print)1176-6328.

5. Gaudiano BA, Dalrymple KL, Zimmerman M. Prevalence and clinical characteristics of psychotic versus nonpsychotic major depression in a general psychiatric outpatient clinic. *Depress Anxiety.* 2009;26(1):54–64. (Print)1091-4269.

6. Kahn JP. *Angst: Origins of Anxiety and Depression.* New York: Oxford University Press; 2013, ISBN:0199796440.

7. Johnson J, Weissman MM, Klerman GL. Service utilization and social morbidity associated with depressive symptoms in the community. *JAMA.* 1992;267(11):1478–1483.

8. Ohayon MM, Schatzberg AF. Prevalence of depressive episodes with psychotic features in the general population. *Am J Psychiatry.* 2002;159(11):1855–1861. (Print)0002-953x.

9. Crebbin K, Mitford E, Paxton R, et al. Drug and alcohol misuse in first episode psychosis: an observational study. *Neuropsychiatr Dis Treat.* 2008;4(2):417–423 [Print].

10. Coryell W. The facets of melancholia. *Acta Psychiatrica Scandinavica.* 2007;115:31–36. ISSN 0001-690X.

11. Coryell W, Leon A, Winokur G. Importance of psychotic features to long-term course in major depressive disorder. *Am J Psychiatry.* 1996;153(4):484–489.

12. Santa Clara CJDS. Melancolia: da antiguidade à modernidade—uma breve análisehistórica. *Mental.* 2009;7: 91–108.

13. Kendler KS. The genealogy of major depression: symptoms and signs of melancholia from 1880 to 1900. *Mol Psychiatry.* 2017;22(11):1539–1553.

14. Kraepelin E. Klinische Psychiatrie. JA Barth, 1899. *Textbook of psychiatry:* London: Macmillan; 1907.

15. Schneider K. Primary and secondary symptoms of schizophrenia (1957). In: Shepperd SHM, editor. *Themes and Variations on European Psychiatry.* Bristol: John Wright & Sons Ltd; 1974:40–4.

16. Kendler KS. The phenomenology of major depression and the representativeness and nature of DSM criteria. *Am J Psychiatry.* 2016;173(8):771–780.

17. American Psychiatric Association. *Diagnostic and Statistical Manual of Mental Disorders (DSM-III®).* American Psychiatric Pub; 1980.

18. Parker G, Fink M, Shorter E, et al. Issues for DSM5: whither melancholia? The case for its classification as a distinct mood disorder. *Am J Psychiatry.* 2010;167:745–747.

19. Rosenthal NE, Sack DA, Gillin JC, et al. Seasonal affective disorder: a description of the syndrome and preliminary findings with light therapy. *Arch Gen Psychiatry.* 1984;41(1):72–80.

20. Harris M, Farquhar F, Healy D, et al. The incidence and prevalence of admissions for melancholia in two cohorts (1875–1924 and 1995–2005). *J Affect Disord.* 2011;134(1–3):45–51.

21. Mcgrath PJ, Khan AY, Trivedi MH, et al. Response to a selective serotonin reuptake inhibitor (citalopram) in major depressive disorder with melancholic features: a STAR*D report. *J Clin Psychiatry.* 2008;69(12):1847–1855.

22. Wigman JT, van Nierop M, Vollebergh WA, et al. Evidence that psychotic symptoms are prevalent in disorders of anxiety and depression, impacting on illness onset, risk, and severity—implications for diagnosis and ultra-high risk research. *Schizophr Bull.* 2012;38(2):247–257. (Print)0586-7614.

23. Maudsley H. *The Pathology of Mind.* London: Macmillan; 1895.

24. Bressan RA. A depressãonaesquizofrenia. *Braz J Psychiatr.* 2000;22:27–30.

25. Zhang N, Wang CX, Wang AX, et al. Time course of depression and one-year prognosis of patients with stroke in Mainland China. *CNS Neurosci Therapeut.* 2012;18(6):475–481. ISSN 1755-5930.

26. Bryan CJ, Rudd MD. Advances in the assessment of suicide risk. *J Clin Psychol.* 2006;62(2):185–200.

27. Parker G, Hadzi-Pavlovic D, Hickie I, et al. Distinguishing psychotic and non-psychotic melancholia. *J Affect Disord.* 1991;22(3):135–148. (Print)0165-0327.

28. Jackson SW. *Melancholia and Depression: From Hippocratic Times to Modern Times.* New Haven, CT: Yale University Press; 1986, ISBN:0300037007.

29. Parker G, Hadzi-Pavlovic D, Roussos J, et al. Non-melancholic depression: the contribution of personality, anxiety and life events to subclassification. *Psychol Med.* 1998;28(5):1209–1219. ISSN 1469u-8978.

30. Brown WA. Treatment response in melancholia. *Acta Psychiatr Scand Suppl.* 2007;433:125–129. (Print)0065-1591.

31. Willeit M, Praschak-Rieder N, Neumeister A, et al. A polymorphism (5-HTTLPR) in the serotonin transporter promoter gene is associated with DSM-IV depression subtypes in seasonal affective disorder. *Mol Psychiatry.* 2003;8(11):942.

32. Akin D, Manier DH, Sanders-Bush E, et al. Signal transduction abnormalities in melancholic depression. *Int J Neuropsychopharmacol.* 2005;8(1):5–16.

33. Hickie I, Naismith S, Ward PB, et al. Reduced hippocampal volumes and memory loss in patients with early-and late-onset depression. *Br J Psychiatry.* 2005;186(3):197–202.
34. Rush AJ, Weissenburger JE. Melancholic symptom features and DSM-IV. *Am J Psychiatry.* 1994;151(4):489.
35. Armitage R. Sleep and circadian rhythms in mood disorders. *Acta Psychiatr Scand Suppl.* 2007;433:104–115. (Print) 0065-1591.
36. Mehl S, Landsberg MW, Schmidt AC, et al. Why do bad things happen to me? Attributional style, depressed mood, and persecutory delusions in patients with schizophrenia. *Schizophr Bull.* 2014;40(6):1338–1346. https://doi.org/10.1093/schbul/sbu040. Epub 2014 Apr 17.
37. Bentall RP, Kinderman P, Kaney S. The self, attributional process and abnormal beliefs: towards a model of persecutory delusions. *Behav Res Ther.* 1994;32:331–341.
38. Veras AB, Cougo S, Meira F, et al. Schizophrenia dissection by five anxiety and depressive subtype comorbidities: clinical implications and evolutionary perspective. *Psychiatry Res.* 2017;257:172–178.
39. Khan AY, Carrithers J, Preskorn SH, et al. Clinical and demographic factors associated with DSM-IV melancholic depression. *Ann Clin Psychiatry.* 2006;18(2):91–98 [Print].
40. Dennis B, Nelson JC, Quinlan DM. Personality traits and disorder in depression. *Am J Psychiatry.* 1981;138:1601.
41. Titley WB. Prepsychotic personality of patients with involutional melancholia. *Arch Neurol Psychiatry.* 1936;36(1):19–33.
42. Von Zerssen D. Melancholic and manic types of personality as premorbid structures in affective disorders. In: Mundt C, Goldstein MJ, Hahlweg K, et al., eds. *Interpersonal Factors in the Origin and Course of Affective Disorders.* London: Gaskell; 1996:65–85.
43. Lichstein PR. The medical interview. In: Walker HK, Hall WD, Hurst JW, eds. *Clinical Methods: The History, Physical, and Laboratory Examinations.* 3rd ed. Boston, MA: Butterworths; 1990.
44. Coentre R, Silva-Dos-Santos A, Talina MC. Retrospective study on structural neuroimaging in first-episode psychosis. *Peer J.* 2016;4:e2069. (Print) 2167–8359.
45. Bürgy M. Study of delusional depression: drive, dynamics, therapy. *Neurol Psychiatry Brain Res.* 2018;30:117–124.
46. Bürgy M. Delusional depression: diagnostics, phenomenology and therapy. *Der Nervenarzt.* 2017;88(5):529–537.
47. Addington J, Shah H, Liu L, et al. Reliability and validity of the Calgary Depression Scale for Schizophrenia (CDSS) in youth at clinical high risk for psychosis. *Schizoph Res.* 2014;153:64–67.
48. Ostergaard SD, Rothschild AJ, Flint AJ, et al. Rating scales measuring the severity of psychotic depression. *Acta Psychiatr Scand.* 2015;132(5):335–344. ISSN 0001-690x.
49. Fedorová S, Blažková M, Humpolíček P, et al. Cognitive impairment in major depressive disorder and severe depressive episode with psychotic symptoms. *Eur Psychiatry.* 2017;41:S143–S144.
50. Schulz P, Macher JP. The clinical pharmacology of depressive states. *Dialogues Clin Neurosci.* 2002;4(1):47–56. (Print)1294-8322.
51. Bolwig TG, Madsen TM. Electroconvulsive therapy in melancholia: the role of hippocampal neurogenesis. *Acta Psychiatr Scand Suppl.* 2007;433:130–135. (Print)0065-1591.
52. Meyers BS, Klimstra SA, Gabriele M, et al. Continuation treatment of delusional depression in older adults. *Am J Geriatr Psychiatry.* 2001;9(4):415–422.
53. Burcusa SL, Iacono WG. Risk for recurrence in depression. *Clin Psychol Rev.* 2007;27(8):959–985 [Print].
54. Buckman JE, Underwood A, Clarke K, et al. Risk factors for relapse and recurrence of depression in adults and how they operate: a four-phase systematic review and meta-synthesis. *Clin Psychol Rev.* 2018;64:13.
55. Gournellis R. Tournikioti K1, Touloumi G, et al. Psychotic (delusional) depression and suicidal attempts: a systematic review and meta-analysis. *Acta Psychiatr Scand.* 2018;137(1):18–29. ISSN 0001-690X.
56. Xin LM, Chen L, Su YA, et al. Risk factors for recent suicide attempts in major depressive disorder patients in China: results from a national study. *Front Psychiatry.* 2018;9:300. (Print)1664-0640.
57. Coryell W, Pfohl B, Zimmerman M. The clinical and neuroendocrine features of psychotic depression. *J Nerv Mental Dis.* 1984;172(9):521–528.
58. Lyness JM, Conwell Y, Nelson JC. Suicide attempts in elderly psychiatric inpatients. *J Am Geriatr Soc.* 1992;40(4):320–324.
59. Isometsä E, Henriksson M, Aro H, et al. Suicide in psychotic major depression. *J Affect Disord.* 1994;31(3):187–191.

60. Freeman D, Garety PA, Kuipers E, et al. Acting on persecutory delusions: the importance of safety seeking. *Behav Res Ther.* 2007;45(1):89–99.
61. Park SC, Lee HY, Sakong JK, et al. Distinctive clinical correlates of psychotic major depression: the CRESCEND study. *Psychiatry Investig.* 2014;11(3):281–289. (Print)1738-3684.
62. Rush AJ, Giles DE, Schlesser MA, et al. The dexamethasone suppression test in patients with mood disorders. *J Clin Psychiatry.* 1996;57(10):470–484. (Print)0160-6689.
63. Fink M, Bolwig TG, Parker G, et al. Melancholia: restoration in psychiatric. *Act Psychiatr Scand.* 2007;115(2):89–92.
64. Parker G, Mccraw S. The properties and utility of the CORE measure of melancholia. *J Affect Disord.* 2017;207:128–135.
65. Thase ME. Depression and sleep: pathophysiology and treatment. *Dialogues Clin Neurosci.* 2006;8(2):217–226. (Print)1294-8322.
66. Spanemberg L, Caldieraro MA, Vares EA, et al. Biological differences between melancholic and non-melancholic depression subtyped by the CORE measure. *Neuropsychiatr Dis Treat.* 2014;10:1523–1531. (Print)1176-6328.
67. Maes M, Ringel K, Kubera M, et al. Increased autoimmune activity against 5-HT: a key component of depression that is associated with inflammation and activation of cell-mediated immunity, and with severity and staging of depression. *J Affect Disord.* 2012;136(3):386–392.
68. Shelton RC, Miller AH. Eating ourselves to death (and despair): the contribution of adiposity and inflammation to depression. *Prog Neurobiol.* 2010;91(4):275–299. (Print)0301-0082.
69. Sarrias MJ, Artigas F, Martínez E, et al. Decreased plasma serotonin in melancholic patients: a study with clomipramine. *Biol Psychiatry.* 1987;22(12):1429–1438. (Print)0006-3223.
70. Soriano-Mas C, Hernández-Ribas R, Pujol J, et al. Cross-sectional and longitudinal assessment of structural brain alterations in melancholic depression. *Biol Psychiatry.* 2011;69(4):318–325.
71. Parker G, Mcclure G, Paterson A. Melancholia and catatonia: disorders or specifiers? *Curr Psychiatry Rep.* 2015;17(1):536.
72. Shankman SA, Sarapas C, Klein DN. The effect of pre- vs. post-reward attainment on EEG asymmetry in melancholic depression. *Int J Psychophysiol.* 2011;79(2):287–295. (Print)0167-8760.
73. Domschke K. Clinical and molecular genetics of psychotic depression. *Schizophr Bull.* 2013;39(4):766–775 [Print].
74. Maier W, Lichtermann D, Minges J, et al. Schizoaffective disorder and affective disorders with mood-incongruent psychotic features: keep separate or combine? Evidence from a family study. *Am J Psychiatry.* 1992;149(12):1666–1673. (Print)0002-953x.
75. Winokur G, Scharfetter C, Angst J. A family study of psychotic symptomatology in schizophrenia, schizoaffective disorder, unipolar depression, and bipolar disorder. *Eur Arch Psychiatry Neurol Sci.* 1985;234(5):295–298. (Print)0175-758x.
76. Domschke K, Lawford B, Young R, et al. Dysbindin (DTNBP1)—a role in psychotic depression? *J Psychiatr Res.* 2011;45(5):588–595.
77. Hamshere ML, Bennett P, Williams N, et al. Genomewide linkage scan in schizoaffective disorder: significant evidence for linkage at 1q42 close to DISC1, and suggestive evidence at 22q11 and 19p13. *Arch Gen Psychiatry.* 2005;62(10):1081–1088. (Print)0003-990x.
78. Klaassen RM, Heins M, Luteijn LB, et al. Depressive symptoms are associated with (sub)clinical psychotic symptoms in patients with non-affective psychotic disorder, siblings and healthy controls. *Psychol Med.* 2013;43(4):747–756.

CHAPTER 7

Bipolar I Mania and Atypical Depression

Mariana Bonotto Mallmann ◾ Fabiana Leão Lopes ◾ André Barciela Veras

Abstract

Atypical depression may be the most common specific subtype of depression. Sensitivity to social rejection is a core symptom. It is generally chronic, variably intense, with reverse vegetative symptoms, and with a reactive mood—all of these in contrast to acute episodes of melancholic depression. Bipolar I disorder requires one or more episodes of mania (commonly including delusions of grandeur), and typically includes atypical depression as well. Medications for treatment and prevention of mania do not eliminate risk and consequences of atypical depression. Careful diagnosis of both conditions is important for optimal outcomes. Augmentation with selective serotonin reuptake inhibitor antidepressants is often beneficial, after careful attention to potential risks and benefits. Although existing data do no offer a clearly defined biological link suggesting that Bipolar I mania is a psychotic form of atypical depression, there could be a phase-shift relationship between these two affective conditions.

KEYWORDS

Atypical depression	Bipolar disorder	Bipolar I
Personality disorder	Mania	Psychotic disorder

Introduction

Atypical depression (AD) is a common condition in clinical practice.[1,2] Instead of the classical symptoms of melancholic depression, AD is characterized by hyperphagia, hypersomnia, and rejections sensitivity. Exacerbations are often triggered by perceived interpersonal slights and heightened social rejection.[3] Rejection sensitivity, though painful, may once have been a useful social instinct that encouraged inoffensive behavior and thus promoted social harmony.[4]

AD is the most common type of clinical depression in bipolar I disorder (previously known as manic depression). This serious disorder frequently leads to hospitalization, and, when untreated, can have long-term effects on career and social life. AD may be ongoing between manic periods, but episodic and of variable intensity. AD can also occur without mania or be associated with such other syndromes as personality disorders and panic anxiety. Early and accurate recognition and treatment of AD and bipolar I disorder are important for best clinical practice.

TABLE 7.1 ■ Diagnostic Criteria: Major Depressive Disorder

DSM5 296.2/296.3 (F32/F33)

A. Five (or more) of the following symptoms have been present during the same 2-week period and represent a change from previous functioning; at least one of the symptoms is either (1) depressed mood or (2) loss of interest or pleasure.
   1. Depressed mood most of the day, nearly every day, as indicated by either subjective report (e.g., feels sad, empty, hopeless) or observation made by others (e.g., appears tearful). (Note: In children and adolescents, can be irritable mood.)
   2. Markedly diminished interest or pleasure in all, or almost all, activities most of the day, nearly every day (as indicated by either subjective account or observation).
   3. Significant weight loss when not dieting or weight gain (e.g., a change of more than 5% of body weight in a month), or decrease or increase in appetite nearly every day.
   4. Insomnia or hypersomnia nearly every day.
   5. Psychomotor agitation or retardation nearly every day (observable by others, not merely subjective feelings of restlessness or being slowed down).
   6. Fatigue or loss of energy nearly every day.
   7. Feelings of worthlessness or excessive or inappropriate guilt (which may be delusional) nearly every day (not merely self-reproach or guilt about being sick).
   8. Diminished ability to think or concentrate, or indecisiveness, nearly every day (either by subjective account or as observed by others).
   9. Recurrent thoughts of death (not just fear of dying), recurrent suicidal ideation without a specific plan, or a suicide attempt or a specific plan for committing suicide.

B. The symptoms cause clinically significant distress or impairment in social, occupational, or other important areas of functioning.

C. The episode is not attributable to the physiologic effects of a substance or to another medical condition.

D. The occurrence of the major depressive episode is not better explained by schizoaffective disorder, schizophrenia, schizophreniform disorder, delusional disorder, or other specified and unspecified schizophrenia spectrum and other psychotic disorders.

E. There has never been a manic episode or a hypomanic episode.

Major Depressive Disorder (page 160—code 296.2/296.3, F32, F33).
American Psychiatric Association. Depressive disorders. In: *Diagnostic and Statistical Manual of Mental Disorders*. 5th ed. 2013. https://doi.org/10.1176/appi.books.9780890425596.dsm04.

This chapter addresses clinical characteristics and associations of AD, in order to facilitate diagnosis and treatment, and clarify relationships to psychotic manifestations (Table 7.1).

Atypical Depression

The term AD was initially chosen to contrast classical melancholic depression (Chapter 6) with another depressive syndrome that has a specific symptom profile of reversed vegetative symptoms.[5,6] The more classical (melancholic, agitated, "endogenous") presentations of depression were the norm at a time when depression was infrequently diagnosed in outpatients, and almost never in adolescents or younger adults.

Importantly, the word "atypical" had also been used to describe depressive presentations that were out of the ordinary. But as the concept of AD has evolved over the years, it no longer connotes an uncommon or unusual clinical presentation. Indeed, the use of AD as a specific type of depression was codified in clinical psychiatry with the publication of the *Diagnostic and Statistical Manual for Mental Disorders Fourth Edition* (DSM-IV).[7]

DSM-IV introduced formal criteria for "atypical features" as a modifier for both major depression and dysthymia, and these criteria are retained in DSM5.[3] When there is a diagnosis of major depression or dysthymia, a diagnosis of AD requires the presence of the DSM5 specifiers for atypical features,[8] when the features predominate during the majority of days of the current or most recent major depressive episode or of a persistent depressive disorder. Clinically, AD is common both in unipolar depressions and, together with mania, in bipolar disorders.

DIAGNOSTIC CRITERIA

According to the DSM5, the criteria for depressive disorders with atypical features include the following (Table 7.2).

As noted above, mood reactivity is a main symptom of AD. One study showed that the most common symptom reported by patients with AD was mood reactivity, at 89% to 90%, but other symptoms (rejection sensitivity, leaden paralysis, and hypersomnia) were nearly as common, 78% to 89%.[9] This has led to further work, suggesting that AD could be diagnosed with comparable validity if only three of the first five inclusion criteria (including mood reactivity) are present, or just two of the four criteria if mood reactivity is excluded.[10]

It has also been proposed that pathologic sensitivity to perceived interpersonal rejection is a core feature of AD. Rejection sensitivity can lead to significant social or occupational impairment.[11] Understanding the full clinical picture of AD includes awareness of mood and physiological and psychological symptoms. With that perspective, AD typically persists or recurs in varying degree over an extended time scale.

PREVALENCE, COURSE, AND COMORBIDITY

Estimates of AD prevalence in depressed patients range from 15.7% to 43%.[9,10,12-15] In community samples, the prevalence of AD based on reversed neurovegetative symptoms was in the range of 11% to 16% and about 6.5% of people with major depression met the criteria for AD.[1,2] Seasonal

---

TABLE 7.2 ■ **Specifiers for Depressive Disorders: Atypical Depression**

DSM5 296 (ICD10 F32)

Specify if:
With atypical features: This specifier can be applied when these features predominate during the majority of days of the current or most recent major depressive episode or persistent depressive disorder.

A. Mood reactivity (i.e., mood brightens in response to actual or potential positive events).

B. Two (or more) of the following:
  1. Significant weight gain or increase in appetite.
  2. Hypersomnia.
  3. Leaden paralysis (i.e., heavy, leaden feelings in arms or legs).
  4. A long-standing pattern of interpersonal rejection sensitivity (not limited to episodes of mood disturbance) that results in significant social or occupational impairment.

C. Criteria are not met for "With melancholic features" or "With catatonia" during the same episode.

Specifiers for Depressive Disorder: **atypical features** (page 185–186—code 296.2/296.3, F32, F33).
American Psychiatric Association. Depressive disorders. In: *Diagnostic and Statistical Manual of Mental Disorders*. 5th ed. 2013. https://doi.org/10.1176/appi.books.9780890425596.dsm04.

affective disorder (SAD) and AD have overlapping symptom pictures, and may reflect differing presentations of the same underlying pathophysiology.[16]

AD is associated with a range of emotional, physical, sexual, financial, and catastrophic hardships across the life span. This painful course of AD has important implications for health care utilization and costs. AD's commonplace psychiatric comorbidities can include panic anxiety, social anxiety, eating disorders, and substance-related disorders[17] along with such self-reported diagnoses as schizophrenia and autism spectrum disorders. Whether or not AD occurs with a broader mood disorder, there is increased risk of suicidal thought, suicide attempts, medically significant weight gain, substance use, social withdrawal, and interpersonal problems with family members, intimate partners, schoolmates, teachers, coworkers, or employers.[18]

Individuals with AD are also more likely to experience socioeconomic disadvantage than depressed individuals without AD.[19] The combination of AD and bipolar disorder increases the risk of substance abuse and somatization disorder.[9,12,20,21] Each of these other diagnoses, life events, and interpersonal factors most likely contribute to the adverse consequences of AD.

AD is more commonly diagnosed in women, especially younger women.[18,19,22,23] Women have a younger age of onset, more depressive episodes, greater functional impairment,[14,24–26] and more adverse life events such as psychological trauma.[18,27] As with some other psychiatric diagnoses, it is possible that women are on average more likely than men to reveal emotional distress or to seek help.

ATYPICAL DEPRESSION AND BIPOLAR DISORDER

Perhaps most importantly for psychosis comorbidity, patients with AD are more likely to experience a lifetime bipolar I manic episode.[19] In discussing bipolar disorders, it is important that the older manic-depressive diagnostic name required episodes of true mania, and roughly corresponds to what is now called bipolar I disorder. In addition, milder degrees of increased mood variation are considered bipolar II. Some authors consider AD as part of this broadly defined "bipolar spectrum."[13,20,28,29] Other studies suggest a considerable overlap of AD manifestations with borderline personality disorder and with bipolar spectrum disorder.[30–32] When adopting moderately strict criteria for bipolar spectrum disorders based on DSM-IV, 24% of AD patients could be classified as bipolar,[33] while broader bipolar criteria produced a prevalence of 72% in another AD sample (major depression with atypical features).[20] Furthermore, studies of bipolar disorders have found comorbid AD with prevalence rates as high as two-thirds.[30,34,35] A Polish cross-sectional study of depression found a significantly higher frequency of AD symptoms (hypersomnia and hyperphagia) in the bipolar patients as compared to the unipolar patients.[12]

Importantly, research has found that those with AD have significantly higher rates of bipolar I disorder than those without atypical features.[25] AD-diagnosed patients seen in clinical practice had a higher family history prevalence of bipolar disorder compared to those without AD.[25] AD symptoms may also be more pronounced in those patients with bipolar disorder.[25] Male bipolar patients compared with unipolar depressed ones had significantly more episodes of AD (OR 2.82).[36] Another study compared bipolar depression patients to unipolar depression patients and found a significant increase in state rejection sensitivity when depressed.[37] Increased rejection sensitivity when depressed further supports AD-like bipolar depression over unipolar depression. Another piece of evidence for this is that bipolar I subjects report increased seasonal changes in social activity and in weight. Simonsen et al.[38] also observed that bipolar subjects slept significantly more throughout the year, and slept for a mean of 1.8 hours more in winter than in summer.

ATYPICAL DEPRESSION AND PERSONALITY DISORDERS

AD is also associated with certain personality disorders. The tendency to anticipate rejection and failure, and the consequent tendency to give up easily when frustrated, is a characteristic of avoidant personality (passive, timid, submissive, easily hurt). Borderline personalities are emotionally unstable, self-destructively impulsive, chronically bored or angry, with constantly shifting moods. Histrionic personalities are flamboyant, self-dramatizing, self-centered, and emotionally shallow. These personality descriptions reflect different styles of coping with the rejection sensitivity and mood reactivity of AD. However, a narrow focus on associated personality disorders lead to diagnostic omission. Research suggests that AD may be a missed diagnosis in personality disorders such as borderline, histrionic, or avoidant.[33,39] One reason for that is that the longer an episode of depression lasts—and AD can be lifelong—the more it begins to look like personality, with the rejection sensitivity of AD appearing to be merely a personality trait rather than a concurrent emotional trait. Although AD improves with medication, an associated personality disorder untreated by psychotherapy might moderate, but would likely continue.

Bipolar I Mania

Fluctuations in mood are common in life, particularly when faced by stressful events. Nevertheless, when mood swings are striking and persistent, and result in notable distress or impairment, there could be an underlying affective disorder. As above, the bipolar spectrum disorders reflect the extent and severity of mood elevation, from unipolar to bipolar II to bipolar I. Individuals with unipolar disorder present with depressive episodes only, and those with bipolar II or I disorder show increasingly pronounced episodes of mood elevation.[40]

In the DSM-5,[3] the modern bipolar I differs from the classic manic depression only to the extent that neither psychosis nor the lifetime experience of major depression is required. However, the vast majority of individuals whose symptoms meet full criteria for a true manic episode do also experience major depression during the course of their lives. Manic episodes are frequently preceded by or followed by hypomanic or major depressive episodes. Manic episodes commonly include grandiose delusions, and sometimes include other delusions and auditory hallucinations.

The "bipolar depressive" phases of bipolar I disorder typically have AD symptoms and course. Bipolar depression and AD are characterized by mood reactivity and often by the atypical physical symptoms of oversleeping and overeating. Especially when milder, bipolar depressive symptoms can be difficult to distinguish from depression with atypical features. Some research suggests that a family history of bipolar disorder is more likely in depressed people with the atypical symptoms of leaden paralysis and oversleeping. Hypersomnia is an important clinical feature of both bipolar depression[41] and AD. In another study, leaden paralysis, increased appetite, weight gain, and rejection sensitivity (common symptoms in AD) were more often seen in bipolar patients (Table 7.3).[12]

Atypical Depression and Psychosis Risk

Some studies have explored the core AD symptom of rejection sensitivity in patients with psychotic disorders. Rejection sensitivity is a trait characterized by increased concern about, and therefore expectation of, interpersonal rejection.[42] Rejection sensitivity also leads to rejection attribution bias.[43] In order to avoid rejection, rejection sensitivity thus leads many people to strive for inoffensiveness, including through small-scale helpfulness.

Rejection sensitivity may be associated with psychosis vulnerability, throughout the psychosis continuum,[44–46] including along the schizophrenia spectrum.[46] Although little research has

TABLE 7.3 ■ Diagnostic Criteria: Bipolar I Disorder

DSM5 296.4 (ICD-10 F31.1)

For a diagnosis of bipolar I disorder, it is necessary to meet the following criteria for a manic episode. The manic episode may have been preceded by and may be followed by hypomanic or major depressive episodes.

Manic Episode

A. **Distinct period of abnormally and persistently elevated, expansive, or irritable mood and abnormally and persistently increased goal-directed behavior or energy, lasting at least 1 week and present most of the day, nearly every day (or any duration if hospitalization is necessary).**

B. **During the period of mood disturbance and increased energy or activity, three (or more) of the following symptoms (four if the mood is only irritable) are present to a significant degree and represent a noticeable change from usual behavior.**
   1. Inflated self-esteem or grandiosity
   2. Decreased need for sleep (e.g., feels rested after only 3 hours of sleep)
   3. More talkative than usual or pressure to keep talking
   4. Flight of ideas or subjective experience that thoughts are racing
   5. Distractibility (i.e., attention too easily drawn to unimportant or irrelevant external stimuli), as reported or observed.
   6. Increase in goal-directed activity (either socially, at work or school, or sexually) or psychomotor agitation (i.e., purposeless non-goal-directed activity).
   7. Excessive involvement in activities that have a high potential for painful consequences (e.g., engaging in unrestrained buying sprees, sexual indiscretions, or foolish business investments).

C. The mood disturbance is sufficiently severe to cause marked impairment in social or occupational functioning or to necessitate hospitalization to prevent harm to self or others, or there are psychotic features.

D. The episode is not attributable to the physiologic effects of a substance (e.g., a drug of abuse, a medication, other treatment) or to another medical condition.

Note: A full manic episode that emerges during antidepressant treatment (e.g., medication, electroconvulsive therapy) but persists at a fully syndromal level beyond the physiologic effect of that treatment is sufficient evidence for a manic episode and, therefore, a bipolar I diagnosis.
Note: Criteria A–D constitute a manic episode. At least one lifetime manic episode is required for the diagnosis of bipolar I disorder.

Bipolar I Disorder (page 123—code 296.41, F31).
American Psychiatric Association. Bipolar and related disorders. In: *Diagnostic and Statistical Manual of Mental Disorders*. 5th ed. 2013. https://doi.org/10.1176/appi.books.9780890425596.dsm03.

evaluated psychotic symptoms in AD, one study did report psychotic features in 13.9% of AD patients undergoing electroconvulsive therapy.[47]

Rejection sensitivity is also associated with co-occurring borderline personality disorder among adults with mood disorder[48,49] and elevates the risk for borderline personality,[50] which in turn increases risk for psychotic symptoms.[51] Some authors suggest that rejection sensitivity is a "soft" bipolar II disorder feature, supporting the idea that AD is part of the bipolar spectrum.[33]

Fictional Case

Mia, a 20-year-old Caucasian woman in São Paulo, Brazil, was brought to a psychiatrist by her mother for her quiet demeanor and limited social network, in the context of the mother's medication and psychotherapy for her own bipolar I depression. Mia said that she had no close friends, and no one to talk to at college. She could not figure out how she had ever offended them, and by now kept her distance lest she be rejected or even offend them more. When the class broke up into work teams, Mia never invited anyone, and always waited for someone who needed a partner, or for her concerned professor to assign her one. The mother also reported a recent period of ill-defined hyperactivity that had lasted at least a few days.

At age 13, Mia started having trouble waking up for school, leading to daily wake-up visits from her mother, and an occasional argument. She would often seem sad and lethargic, although she denied it at first. Not unhappy, just not happy, she said then. These depressive episodes often followed some perceived rejection. At that age, her appetite did not increase with depression, but she did have cravings for pasta and chocolates. She would cheer up whenever she received a friendly message online, but it would quickly fade back to depression. And an evolving seasonal component increased the frequency and intensity of depressed mood during the Brazilian winter. This was more evident on a visit to relatives during the Canadian winter.

At home, Mia started to stay in her bedroom watching TV, eating, sleeping, or surfing the web. To reduce her loneliness, she would sometimes sit quietly in a room with family. With her frequently depressed mood and lethargy, Mia had to summon up much more effort to complete her homework, but concentration was a problem, and it took longer to finish her work.

At 15, her teacher passed her on the sidewalk but did not greet her. Mia was sure that she saw her but just did not want to say hello. She thought that the slight was solid evidence of rejection that was somehow her fault, felt immensely hurt, and holed up in her room for hours. Eventually she talked to her mother, but it was 2 days before she had the courage to return to school.

At 18, Mia's appetite increased, she began to gain some extra weight. She was now aware of her continuing social isolation and that a chronic, variable depressed mood continued.

At 20, Mia had a period of about 6 days when she slept very little at university, and some nights not at all. Mia became increasingly preoccupied with a grandiose plan to save the Amazon forest by replanting trees faster than they were lost to fire, forestry, and land-clearing. She believed she had been chosen by God for this special mission to save the world. She started trying to raise money for seedlings, and even bought a one-way airline ticket to visit the forest and convert the locals to her cause. She had no time for food, and lost some weight. Her speech was pressured, and her mood elated and irritable. During this time, she also gambled away her savings in an attempt to raise funds, engaged for the first time in a risky sexual encounter, and missed all of her classes and two exams. Fortunately, her symptoms abated before the process continued further. She had no close friends to notice her changed behavior, and shared very little with her mother. Four months later, she presented for treatment.

How to Interview

The psychiatric interview is undertaken primarily to establish a diagnosis. It includes history-taking and the clinical examination of the mental state. However, the psychiatric interview is much more than a diagnostic process. It also helps to establish rapport between patient and doctor and to educate and motivate the patient.[52] Establishing a therapeutic relationship and a diagnosis allows development of a treatment plan.

The interviewer must discover as much as possible about what the patient thinks and feels. During the clinical interview, information is gathered from what the patient tells the interviewer; critically important clues also come from how the history unfolds. Thus, both the content of the interview (i.e., what the patient says) and the process of the interview (i.e., how the patient says it) offer important routes for understanding the patient's problems. Questions should be phrased in a way that invites patients to talk. For patients not acutely psychotic, open-ended questions tend to allow patients to provide information beyond answers to specific or leading questions.[53]

Interviewing for AD includes recalling differences from endogenous or melancholic depression: reactive mood, reverse vegetative symptoms, and rejection sensitivity.[3,54] Frequently, AD begins early in life and affects women in a higher proportion than men.[9] Effective interview technique includes exploring the age of onset of depressive syndromes, as well as current and recent symptoms. Asking friends and relatives about symptoms and relationships provides useful collateral information.

Guided by specific symptoms, an unofficial semi-structured interview can be useful for assessing AD in bipolar I patients and others.[55] This clinically based approach addresses common AD features, and not all symptoms are required for diagnosis:

ATYPICAL DEPRESSION

1. Over the course of your life, have you often had periods of mild to moderate sadness or depression (not just anxiety)? [yes]
   a. At what age did these begin?
2. Think about those times when you have felt more depressed than usual.
3. At those times, what would happen to your energy level? [decreased]
   a. Would you feel physically lethargic? [yes]
   b. Would the lethargy ever be so bad that you felt like you couldn't get off the couch, even though you knew that you could? [yes]
4. At those times, would your appetite go up or down? [up]
   a. Whether or not your appetite increases when sad, would you have cravings for sweets, chocolate, or carbohydrates? [yes]
5. At those times, if your schedule permitted, would you sleep or want to sleep more hours or less hours than usual? [more]
6. At those times, could you cheer up with a nice conversation, a funny joke, or a good movie? [yes]
   a. Would you stay cheered up, or would it be only temporary? [temporary]
7. Most people don't like feeling rejected.
   a. On the inside, do you think you are more sensitive or less sensitive than others to minor social rejections? [more, or much more]
   b. Can you give an example of some minor slight that would leave you feeling hurt or rejected, but that other people would just brush off?
   c. Here is a hypothetical encounter: You are walking down a sidewalk and pass a close friend who clearly sees you but does not say hello. What would be your first emotion? [hurt] What would be your first explanation of what happened? [somehow offended them]

Fictional Case: Treatment

Based on the history of past and current symptoms, Mia was diagnosed as bipolar I, with an episode of mania, as well as chronic AD. To prevent future manic episodes, she was started on lithium, with blood tests to confirm and adjust dosage in the maintenance range, and education about the importance of medication compliance and periodic blood levels, and about the long-term risks of renal and thyroid complications.

After 4 weeks at a maintenance level of lithium, she started fluoxetine 20 mg qd. About a month later, Mia began to notice improved mood and energy. She found it easier to lose some weight through dieting. About 3 months later, she began to notice a modest improvement in her rejection sensitivity. Later on, buspirone 15 mg twice daily was added to enhance the effect of fluoxetine, and further improvement began after 1 week. For the first few months, she was seen weekly for psychotherapy. This helped her understand that mania, AD, and rejection sensitivity have biological underpinnings that are not her fault, and that had colored her view of the world. Relieved by this thought, she could rethink her approach to social life and studies. Later, there was a period of monthly visits to check blood levels and assess for emerging manic symptoms. Once she was stable, she was seen every 3 months.

Treatment

Treatment and prevention of mania are the first concern in acute bipolar I disorder. Lithium, the first treatment for mania, is generally still considered the best choice. Lithium requires careful attention to blood levels, toxicity, side effects, pregnancy, and suicide risk. Onset of action for acute mania is not immediate, and is further delayed by the need for careful dosing. The risk of such long-term side effects as impaired renal function and hypothyroidism require periodic blood tests to catch emergent problems early. Unlike medications that are designed to interact with specific molecular targets, lithium's effects are distributed across many biological processes and pathways. Treatment response is subject to genetic variation between individuals, and similar genetic variation may influence susceptibility to side effects.[56] Long-term prophylaxis after a first manic episode is important for reducing recurrent episodes, allowing return of normal cognition, and preventing other aspects of illness progression. Lithium may also have some degree of antidepressant and antisuicide benefits.[57] After a first manic episode, 1 year of randomized treatment with lithium was superior to quetiapine, supporting the importance of including lithium in the treatment regimen.[58]

For initial stabilization of a manic episode, including patients started on other medications, addition of olanzapine will often take effect earlier than the other agents.[59] However, long-term maintenance with olanzapine risks weight gain and other side effects. For treatment-resistant cases, and when lithium is contraindicated, many other antimanic medications are used, long including the anticonvulsants valproic acid and carbamazepine, as well as more recent medications. As appropriate, these agents can often be combined with lithium, or used on their own.[60] Sometimes, patients need to try several medications or combinations before finding maximal benefit, and for some side effects that diminish over time.

Depending on the type, severity, comorbidities, and course of the disease, specific addition of neuroleptic, antipsychotic, anticonvulsant, anxiolytic, and such other mood-stabilizing medications as lamotrigine, quetiapine, or lurasidone have been shown useful for reversing acute mania and preventing recurrence of crises.[61] Diagnosis and treatment should also address other conditions that often accompany AD and bipolar I, in particular anxiety disorders and drug or alcohol misuse.

Comorbid panic is quite common, and obsessive-compulsive symptoms less so. Both may need psychotherapeutic treatment and selective serotonin reuptake inhibitors (SSRIs).[62] Fixed-dose q12h clonazepam, gradually tapered to an effective dose, can be more effective for panic when SSRIs are either contraindicated or not sufficiently effective.

Perhaps the most important comorbidity focus in bipolar I disorder is AD and other forms of depression. Chronic or recurrent depression can be a major overall determinant of such adverse clinical outcomes as social and workplace dysfunction, emotional distress, and suicide. However, there are important questions about the risk of antidepressants causing a switch into mania. For an acute bipolar depression, antidepressants show moderate benefit until mood stabilization, making continuation reasonable for a few months. Except for selected cases, longer usage for maintenance may increase risk of phase-shifting.[63] It seems likely that adding an appropriate antidepressant to ongoing and effective antimanic medication poses a lower risk of affective conversion. For example, olanzapine with fluoxetine for bipolar I and II depression were more effective for depression than placebo, fluoxetine, or olanzapine, with no suggestions of mania or increased manic symptoms.[64] Another report similarly shows little affective switch in a larger sample taking a variety of mood stabilizers and antidepressants.[65] The combination of lithium with antidepressants and anticonvulsants may be more effective in preventing AD relapse.

Since AD is chronic and recurrent, antidepressants should be considered, and subjected to a thoughtful risk/benefit analysis that includes attention to mania conversion risk. This should be discussed with patient and family, and antidepressant initiation should initially be followed by frequent appointments. SSRI are the first-line medications for AD and appear to carry less conversion risk than such other AD medications as SNRIs.[66] While bupropion may be similarly safer,[67] it is not specific for AD.

Lamotrigine has been prescribed for its antidepressant effects, and limited clinical experience suggests it may have some benefit for AD and bipolar depression.[68,69] When added to a mood stabilizer in a small study, it was equally effective to citalopram for bipolar depression.[70] However, lamotrigine carries a risk of severe Stevens-Johnson syndrome, especially if the dose is raised too fast, or if a high dose is resumed after a period of noncompliance. Lurasidone is approved for bipolar depression in the United States, and little is yet known about benefits for AD.[71]

Psychotherapy, especially cognitive behavioral therapy (CBT), has been widely used in the treatment of depression, including AD. A study points to a different change in specific depressive symptoms during a 16-week antidepressant (paroxetine) or CBT course of treatment, and showed that both treatments reduced cognitive and suicide symptoms.[72] Cognitive therapy may reduce short-term atypical-vegetative symptoms, and may enhance medication benefits for AD.[8]

Psychosis and Atypical Depression

While a phase shift association of AD with bipolar I raises questions of possible linkage, there is limited data to support a theoretical biological link. However, both AD and bipolar I are associated with serotonergic changes,[73] with certain circadian rhythm genes,[74] and with some intriguing clinical features, suggesting a possible evolutionary connection.[4] For example, some symptoms of AD point to behavioral similarities with mammalian hibernation, while some symptoms of mania suggest hibernation awakening. Along these lines, AD is associated with social withdrawal, energy and resource conservation, and necessary inoffensiveness for the close quarters of hibernation, while Bipolar I mania and its delusions are associated with energetic behaviors to reestablish the personal and wider world after hibernation.

Indeed, limited research suggests that while short days exacerbate AD in winter,[75,76] manic episodes are more common with the lengthening daylight hours of spring.[77] In turn, light therapy helps SAD and AD, while dark therapy and artificially shortened perception of day length may diminish acute mania.[78,79] Similarly, adjunctive melatonin (a hormone which signals darkness) may effect faster and greater improvement in acute mania.[80] Time will tell if genetics and physiology further support this theory.

Summary

Because of the debilitating effects of AD, it is essential to screen for it carefully in bipolar patients. This is often best accomplished after acute mania has abated. Proper AD treatment, in addition to anti-manic treatment, may lead to more improvement, better outcomes, and improved prognosis.

AD is linked to bipolar and personality disorders. The depressive stages of bipolar I disorder are associated with AD, which often constitutes the depressive phase. Bipolar depression and AD have similar symptoms. They are characterized by mood reactivity and often by the atypical physical symptoms of oversleeping and overeating. Rejection sensitivity is found in AD and also in many patients along the psychotic spectrum, including schizophrenia spectrum disorders. Some personality disorders also have rejection sensitivity and mood reactivity. However, AD may be inadvertently misdiagnosed as solely a personality disorder, such as borderline, histrionic, or avoidant. Borderline personality, in particular, may include psychotic symptoms. AD and personality disorders can be concurrent, and while medication is usually helpful for the AD component, personality disorders will likely persist without psychotherapy.

References

1. Horwath E, Johnson J, Weissman MM, et al. The validity of major depression with atypical features based on a community study. *J Affect Disord.* 1992;26(2):117–125.
2. Levitan RD, Lesage A, Parikh SV, et al. Reversed neurovegetative symptoms of depression: a community study of Ontario. *Am J Psychiatr.* 1997;154(7):934–940.
3. American Psychiatric Association. *Diagnostic and Statistical Manual of Mental Disorders.* 5th ed. Arlington, VA: American Psychiatric Pub; 2013.
4. Kahn JP. *Angst: Origins of Anxiety and Depression.* New York: Oxford University Press; 2013.
5. Singh T, Williams K. Atypical depression. *Psychiatry (Edgmont).* 2006;3(4):33–39.
6. West ED, Dally PJ. Effects of iproniazid in depressive syndromes. *Brit Med J.* 1959;1(5136):1491–1494. https://doi.org/10.1136/bmj.1.5136.1491.
7. American Psychiatric Association. *Diagnostic and Statistical Manual of Mental Disorders.* 4th ed. Washington, DC: American Psychiatric Press Inc.; 1994.
8. Łojko D, Rybakowski JK. Atypical depression: current perspectives. *Neuropsychiatric Dis Treat.* 2017;13:2447–2456. https://doi.org/10.2147/NDT.S147317.
9. Angst J, Gamma A, Sellaro R, et al. Toward validation of atypical depression in the community: results of the Zurich cohort study. *J Affect Disord.* 2002;72(2):125–138.
10. Angst J, Gamma A, Benazzi F, et al. Atypical depressive syndromes in varying definitions. *Eur Arch Psychiatr Clin Neurosci.* 2006;256(1):44–54.
11. Parker GB. Atypical depression: a valid subtype? *J Clin Psychiatr.* 2007;68(Suppl 3):18–22.
12. Łojko D, Buzuk G, Owecki M, et al. Atypical features in depression: association with obesity and bipolar disorder. *J Affect Disord.* 2015;185:76–80.
13. Akiskal HS, Benazzi F. Atypical depression: a variant of bipolar II or a bridge between unipolar and bipolar II? *J Affect Disord.* 2005;84(2–3):209–217.
14. Nierenberg AA, Alpert JE, Pava J, et al. Course and treatment of atypical depression. *J Clin Psychiatr.* 1998;59:5–9.
15. Novick JS, Stewart JW, Wisniewski SR, et al. Clinical and demographic features of atypical depression in outpatients with major depressive disorder: preliminary findings from STAR*D. *J Clin Psychiatr.* 2005;66(8):1002–1011.
16. Jurena MF, Cleare J. Superposição entre depressão atípica, doença afetiva sazonal e síndrome da fadiga crônica [Overlap between atypical depression, seasonal affective disorder and chronic fatigue syndrome]. *Rev Bras Psiquiatr.* 2007;29(Suppl 1):S19–S26.
17. Pae CU, Tharwani H, Marks DM, et al. Atypical depression: a comprehensive review. *CNS Drugs.* 2009;23(12):1023–1037.
18. Matza LS, Revicki DA, Davidson JR, et al. Depression with atypical features in the national comorbidity survey: classification, description, and consequences. *Arch General Psychiatr.* 2003;60(8):817–826.
19. Brailean A, Curtis J, Davis K, et al. Characteristics, comorbidities, and correlates of atypical depression: evidence from the UK Biobank Mental Health Survey. *Psychol Med.* 2020;50(7):1129–1138.
20. Perugi G, Akiskal HS, Lattanzi L, et al. The high prevalence of "soft" bipolar (II) features in atypical depression. *Compr Psychiatr.* 1998;39(2):63–71.
21. Posternak MA, Zimmerman M. Partial validation of the atypical features subtype of major depressive disorder. *Arch General Psychiatr.* 2002;59(1):70–76.
22. Lee S, Ng KL, Tsang A. Prevalence and correlates of depression with atypical symptoms in Hong Kong. *Australian N Z J Psychiatr.* 2009;43(12):1147–1154.
23. Angst J, Gamma A, Benazzi F, et al. Melancholia and atypical depression in the Zurich study: epidemiology, clinical characteristics, course, comorbidity and personality. *Acta Psychiatr Scand.* 2007;115(Suppl. 433):72–84. https://doi.org/10.1111/j.1600-0447.2007.00965.x.
24. Agosti V, Stewart JW. Atypical and non-atypical subtypes of depression: comparison of social functioning, symptoms, course of illness, co-morbidity and demographic features. *J Affect Disord.* 2001;65(1):75–79. https://doi.org/10.1016/s0165-0327(00)00251-2.

25. Blanco C, Vesga-López O, Stewart JW, et al. Epidemiology of major depression with atypical features: results from the National Epidemiologic Survey on Alcohol and Related Conditions (NESARC). *J Clin Psychiatr.* 2012;73(2):224–232.

26. Stewart JW, McGrath PJ, Rabkin JG, et al. Atypical depression; a valid clinical entity? *Psychiatr Clin North Am.* 1993;16(3):479–495.

27. Withers AC, Tarasoff JM, Stewart JW. Is depression with atypical features associated with trauma history? *J Clin Psychiatr.* 2013;74(5):500–506.

28. Akiskal HS, Pinto O. The evolving bipolar spectrum: prototypes I, II, III, and IV. *Psychiatr Clin North Am.* 1999;23(3):517–534.

29 Perugi G, Toni C, Travierso MC, et al. The role of cyclothymia in atypical depression: toward, a data-based reconceptualization of the borderline-bipolar II connection. *J Affect Disord.* 2003;73(1–2):87–98.

30. Benazzi F. Prevalence of bipolar II disorder in atypical depression. *Eur Arch Psychiatr Clin Neurosci.* 1999;249(2):62–65.

31. Akiskal HS. Subaffective disorders: dysthymic, cyclothymic and bipolar II disorders in the "borderline" realm. *Psychiatr Clin North Am.* 1981;4(1):25–46.

32. Deltito J, Martin L, Riefkohl J, et al. Do patients with borderline personality disorder belong to the bipolar spectrum? *J Affect Disord.* 2001;67(1–3):221–228.

33. Perugi G, Fornaro M, Akiskal HS. Are atypical depression, borderline personality disorder and bipolar II disorder overlapping manifestations of a common cyclothymic diathesis? *World Psychiatr.* 2011;10(1):45–51.

34. Akiskal HS. The prevalent clinical spectrum of bipolar disorders: beyond DSM IV. *J Clin Psychopharmacol.* 1996;16(2):4S–14S.

35. Angst J, Gamma A, Benazzi F, et al. Toward a redefinition of subthreshold bipolarity: epidemiology and proposed criteria for bipolar II, minor bipolar disorders and hypomania. *J Affect Disord.* 2003;73(1–2):133–146.

36. Rybakowski JK, Suwalska A, Lojko D, et al. Types of depression more frequent in bipolar than in unipolar affective illness: results of the Polish DEP-BI study. *Psychopathology.* 2007;40(3):153–158.

37. Ehnvall A, Mitchell PB, Hadzi-Pavlovic D, et al. Rejection sensitivity and pain in bipolar versus unipolar depression. *Bipolar Disord.* 2014;16(2):190–198. https://doi.org/10.1111/bdi.12147.

38. Simonsen H, Shand AJ, Scott NW, et al. Seasonal symptoms in bipolar and primary care patients. *J Affect Disord.* 2011;132(1–2):200–208.

39. Parker G, Roy K, Mitchell P, et al. Atypical depression: a reappraisal. *Am J Psychiatr.* 2002; 159(9): 1470–1479.

40. Cuellar AK, Johnson SL, Winters R. Distinctions between bipolar and unipolar depression. *Clin Psychol Rev.* 2005;25(3):307–339.

41. Forty L, Smith D, Jones L, et al. Clinical differences between bipolar and unipolar depression. *Br J Psychiatr.* 2008;192(5):388–389. https://doi.org/10.1192/bjp.bp.107.045294.

42. Downey G, Feldman SI. Implications of rejection sensitivity for intimate relationships. *J Pers Soc Psychol.* 1996;70(6):1327–1343.

43. Park A, Jensen-Campbell LA, Miller HL. The effects of peer relational victimization on social cognition: rejection attribution bias or a more generalized sensitivity to social pain? *J Soc Pers Relat.* 2017;34(7):984–1006.

44. Kwapil TR, Brown LH, Silvia PJ, et al. The expression of positive and negative schizotypy in daily life: an experience sampling study. *Psychol Med.* 2012;42(12):2555–2566. https://doi.org/10.1017/S0033291712000827.

45. Morrison AP, French P, Lewis SW, et al. Psychological factors in people at ultra-high risk of psychosis: comparisons with non-patients and associations with symptoms. *Psychol Med.* 2006;36(10):1395–1404.

46. Premkumar P, Dunn AK, Onwumere J, et al. Sensitivity to criticism and praise predicts schizotypy in the non-clinical population: the role of affect and perceived expressed emotion. *Eur Psychiatr.* 2019;55:109–115. https://doi.org/10.1016/j.eurpsy.2018.10.009.

47. Husain MM, McClintock SM, Rush AJ, et al. The efficacy of acute electroconvulsive therapy in atypical depression. *J Clin Psychiatr.* 2008;69(3):406–411.

48. Berenson KR, Downey G, Rafaeli E, et al. The rejection-rage contingency in borderline personality disorder. *J Abnorm Psychol.* 2011;120(3):681.

49. Staebler K, Helbing E, Rosenbach C, et al. Rejection sensitivity and borderline personality disorder. *Clin Psychol Psychother.* 2011;18(4):275–283.

50. Chesin M, Fertuck E, Goodman J, et al. The interaction between rejection sensitivity and emotional maltreatment in borderline personality disorder. *Psychopathology.* 2015;48(1):31–35. https://doi.org/10.1159/000365196.

51. Niemantsverdriet MB, Slotema CW, Blom JD, et al. Hallucinations in borderline personality disorder: prevalence, characteristics and associations with comorbid symptoms and disorders. *Sci Rep.* 2017;7(1):13920. https://doi.org/10.1038/s41598-017-13108-6.

52. Eugene VB, Margot P, Gordon C. The psychiatric interview. In: Stern TA, Fricchione GL, Rosenbaum JF, eds. *Massachusetts General Hospital Handbook of General Hospital Psychiatry.* 6th ed. Boston, MA: Elsevier Health Sciences; 2010;4:25–38.

53. Waldinger R, Jacobson A. The initial psychiatric interview. In: Jacobson JL, Jacobson AM, eds. *Psychiatric Secrets.* 2nd ed. Philadelphia: Hanley & Belfus Inc.; 2001.

54. Stewart JW, McGrath PJ, Quitkin FM, et al. Atypical depression: current status and relevance to melancholia. *Acta Psychiatr Scand.* 2007;115(433):58–71.

55. Kahn JP. *Personal communication;* 2019.

56. Pickard BS. Genomics of lithium action and response. *Focus.* 2019;17(3):308–313. https://doi.org/10.1176/appi.focus.17305.

57. Benard V, Vaiva G, Masson M, et al. Lithium and suicide prevention in bipolar disorder. *L'Encéphale.* 2016;42(3):234–241.

58. Post RM. The new news about lithium: an underutilized treatment in the United States. *Neuropsychopharmacology.* 2018;43(5):1174–1179. https://doi.org/10.1038/npp.2017.238.

59. McIntyre RS, Cohen M, Zhao J, et al. Asenapine in the treatment of acute mania in bipolar I disorder: a randomized, double-blind, placebo-controlled trial. *J Affect Disord.* 2010;122(1–2):27–38. https://doi.org/10.1016/j.jad.2009.12.028.

60. Vieta E, Sanchez-Moreno J. Acute and long-term treatment of mania. *Dialogues Clin Neurosci.* 2008;10(2):165–179.

61. Yatham LN, Kennedy SH, Parikh SV, et al. Canadian Network for Mood and Anxiety Treatments (CANMAT) and International Society for Bipolar Disorders (ISBD) 2018 guidelines for the management of patients with bipolar disorder. *Bipolar Disord.* 2018;20(2):97–170. https://doi.org/10.1111/bdi.12609.

62. Ballenger JC, Davidson JR, Lecrubier Y, et al. Consensus statement on post- traumatic stress disorder from the International Consensus Group on Depression and Anxiety. *J Clin Psychiatr.* 2000;61(Suppl 5):60–66.

63. Goodwin GM, Anderson I, Arango C, et al. ECNP consensus meeting. Bipolar depression. Nice, March 2007. *Eur Neuropsychopharmacol.* 18(7):535–549.

64. Amsterdam JD, Shults J. Comparison of fluoxetine, olanzapine, and combined fluoxetine plus olanzapine initial therapy of bipolar type I and type II major depression-lack of manic induction. *J Affect Disord.* 2005;87(1):121–130. https://doi.org/10.1016/j.jad.2005.02.018.

65. Sachs GS, Nierenberg AA, Calabrese JR, et al. Effectiveness of adjunctive antidepressant treatment for bipolar depression. *New Engl J Med.* 2007;356(17):1711–1722. https://doi.org/10.1056/NEJMoa064135.

66. Leverich GS, Altshuler LL, Frye MA, et al. Risk of switch in mood polarity to hypomania or mania in patients with bipolar depression during acute and continuation trials of venlafaxine, sertraline, and bupropion as adjuncts to mood stabilizers. *Am J Psychiatr.* 2006;163(2):232–239. https://doi.org/10.1176/appi.ajp.163.2.232.

67. Pacchiarotti I, Bond DJ, Baldessarini RJ, et al. The International Society for Bipolar Disorders (ISBD) task force report on antidepressant use in bipolar disorders. *Am J Psychiatr.* 2013;170(11):1249–1262.

68. Reid JG, Gitlin MJ, Altshuler LL. Lamotrigine in psychiatric disorders. *J Clin Psychiatr.* 2013;74(7):675–684.

69. Miller JM, Kustra RP, Vuong A, et al. Depressive symptoms in epilepsy. *Drugs.* 2008;68(11):1493–1509. https://doi.org/10.2165/00003495-200868110-00003.

70. Schaffer A, Zuker P, Levitt A. Randomized, double-blind pilot trial comparing lamotrigine versus citalopram for the treatment of bipolar depression. *J Affect Disord.* 2006;96(1–2):95–99. https://doi.org/10.1016/j.jad.2006.05.023.

71. Keks NA, Hope J, Castle D. Lurasidone: an antipsychotic with antidepressant effects in bipolar depression? *Australas Psychiatr.* 2016;24(3):289–291. https://doi.org/10.1177/1039856216641309.

72. Fournier JC, DeRubeis RJ, Hollon SD, et al. Differential change in specific depressive symptoms during antidepressant medication or cognitive therapy. *Behav Res Ther.* 2013;51(7):392–398. https://doi.org/10.1016/j.brat.2013.03.010.

73. Geoffroy PA, Lajnef M, Bellivier F, et al. Genetic association study of circadian genes with seasonal pattern in bipolar disorders. *Sci Rep.* 2015;5:10232. https://doi.org/10.1038/srep10232.

74. Yeim S, Boudebesse C, Etain B, et al. Circadian markers and genes in bipolar disorder. *L'Encephale.* 2015;41(4 Suppl 1):S38–S44. https://doi.org/10.1016/S0013-7006(15)30005-1.

75. Booker JM, Hellekson CJ. Prevalence of seasonal affective disorder in Alaska. *Am J Psychiatr.* 1992;149(9):1176–1182.

76. Rosen LN, Targum SD, Terman M, et al. Prevalence of seasonal affective disorder at four latitudes. *Psychiatr Res.* 1990;31(2):131–144. https://doi.org/10.1016/0165-1781(90)90116-m.

77. Geoffroy PA, Bellivier F, Scott J, et al. Seasonality and bipolar disorder: a systematic review, from admission rates to seasonality of symptoms. *J Affect Disord.* 2014;168:210–223. https://doi.org/10.1016/j.jad.2014.07.002.

78. Barbini B, Benedetti F, Colombo C, et al. Dark therapy for mania: a pilot study. *Bipolar Disord.* 2005;7(1):98–101. https://doi.org/10.1111/j.1399-5618.2004.00166.x.

79. Henriksen TE, Skrede S, Fasmer OB, et al. Blue-blocking glasses as additive treatment for mania: a randomized placebo-controlled trial. *Bipolar Disord.* 2016;18(3):221–232. https://doi.org/10.1111/bdi.12390.

80. Moghaddam HS, Bahmani S, Bayanati S, et al. Efficacy of melatonin as an adjunct in the treatment of acute mania: a double-blind and placebo-controlled trial. *Int Clin Psychopharmacol.* 2020;35(2):81–88. https://doi.org/10.1097/YIC.0000000000000298.

CHAPTER 8

Substance Use Psychosis

Julia Sasiadek   Darby J.E. Lowe   Sarah-Maude Rioux
Tony P. George

Abstract

Substance use disorders (SUDs) are commonly observed in individuals with schizophrenia and related disorders. This chapter reviews the comorbidity between psychotic disorders and SUDs, including etiology, assessment, and treatment. We examine the complexity of substance-induced psychosis and the risk of developing schizophrenia or related disorders. The chapter reviews the impact of individual substances on schizophrenia and the possibility of developing a substance-induced psychosis. The substances reviewed include: alcohol, cannabis, tobacco, hallucinogens, cocaine, amphetamines, and opioids. Afterward we discuss evidence-based approaches to pharmacologic and behavioral treatments for SUDs in psychotic patients, with a focus on schizophrenia. We also discuss the integration of SUD treatment into mental health settings. Given the rates of SUDs and impact on the onset and course of illness in psychotic disorders, treatment of SUDs should be a priority for clinicians working with psychotic patients.

KEYWORDS

Psychosis	Schizophrenia	Substance Use Disorder
Addiction	Antipsychotic	Treatment

Introduction

Schizophrenia is a complex mental disorder that affects nearly 1% of people worldwide and is one of the top 15 leading causes of disability (WHO). Substance use disorder (SUD) comorbidities are commonly seen in individuals with schizophrenia, with lifetime SUDs affecting 47% of patients.[1] SUDs are 4.6 times more common in people with schizophrenia compared to the general population, and males as well as people with lower levels of education are at an increased risk. A dual diagnosis of substance use in schizophrenia complicates the course of treatment and in many cases is associated with poorer outcomes including increased psychotic symptoms, more cognitive impairment, and poorer treatment compliance,[2] including nonadherence to antipsychotic medications, which is a common cause of psychotic symptom relapse and hospitalization.[3,4] More recent studies have identified the risk of substance-induced psychosis and development into schizophrenia, especially in cannabis use disorder.[5]

Fictional Case

Ms. AB is a 19-year-old white female college student who was admitted to the hospital in an acutely psychotic and agitated state. She is in her second year and has become increasingly isolated and bizarre. She started smoking marijuana at the age of 17, and since entering college her pot use has been daily.

In the past month, her roommate observed that she would lock herself in their room, and the room smelled of pot. She has become increasingly suspicious of the other students in her dorm, and she told her Resident Assistant that she felt the other students were stealing from her and trying to poison her. The Dean of Students called her parents and the police, and she was brought to the emergency department.

Fortunately, Ms. AB recognized her cannabis use disorder and entered drug treatment and continued her antipsychotic medication. Within 3 months, her psychosis had cleared and she returned to college.

Theories to Explain Substance Use Disorder Comorbidity: Self-Medication Versus Addiction Vulnerability Hypothesis

Some individuals may be more predisposed to developing an SUD, as well as to developing psychotic disorders.[6,7] The addiction vulnerability hypothesis outlines preexisting vulnerabilities, such as impulsivity, genetic predisposition, epigenetic states, and overlapping neurobiology that bias an individual to not only mental illness but also problematic substance use.[8,9] Moreover, the presence of a mental illness itself is a vulnerability factor for substance use, despite the heterogeneity across comorbidities.[10,11] For example, dysfunctional hippocampal and frontal cortex functioning leading to dysregulated dopaminergic and glutamatergic signaling has been hypothesized to underpin schizophrenia. These abnormalities mimic the reinforcing effects of long-term substance use, as well as facilitate reduced inhibitory control over substance use behavior, placing those with schizophrenia at a vulnerability to the development of an SUD.[8]

The self-medication hypothesis describes how individuals use substances due to dysfunctional self-regulatory tendencies and affective states.[12,13] Individuals medicate the distress and pain associated with "self-regulation" difficulties that are prominent in those with mental illness, such as general self-care, emotion regulation, self-esteem, and interpersonal difficulties.[13] When an individual's distress becomes heightened and he/she experiences emotional dysregulation, substances are more likely to be used to mitigate the feeling due to lack of coping skills, prompting a vulnerability to "self-medication."[12] Alternatively, the theory that substance use directly causes schizophrenia has minimal evidence; however, substances promote much more severe presentations of the disorder and disorder-like episodes.[14,15]

Although the addiction vulnerability hypothesis carries more neurobiological support, the self-medication hypothesis also contributes to our understanding of substance use co-occurring with psychosis. The relief that is associated with substance use is not a true therapeutic effect, but rather a temporary and immediate relief that replaces one's absent self-regulatory and coping processes. The perception of self-medication is more of a driving influence than actual improvement of symptoms.[16]

The initial relief of one's affective state positively reinforces substance use behavior, eventually leading to an allostatic state in which a neurobiological affect deficit is produced (Fig. 8.1).[17] This deficit occurs due to physiologic changes, such as decreased dopamine, endogenous opioid peptides, serotonin and increased dynorphin, as well as decreased GABA and neuropeptide Y, and increased corticotrophin releasing factor (CRF).[18] Koob has conceptualized addiction into a theory that involves a binge and intoxication stage, a withdrawal and negative affect stage, and a preoccupation and anticipation stage, all of which are fueled by negative reinforcement.[19] Negative reinforcement, which is the removal of an aversive stimulus by substance use, maintains addiction.

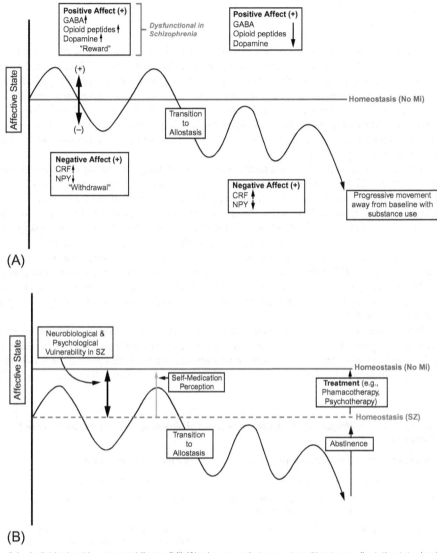

Fig. 8.1 Individuals without mental illness (MI) (**A**) who use substances transition to an allostatic state, leading to neurobiological changes that induce a continuous reduction in positive affect that is associated with further use in attempts to regain original homeostatic levels. Individuals with schizophrenia (SZ) (**B**) already have a lowered set point for positive and negative hedonic homeostasis and dysregulated reward systems, promoting addiction vulnerability, as substances are used in attempts to normalize an already altered (reduced) set point. Addiction in schizophrenia patients is associated with a similar transition to an allostatic state but with an even lower homeostatic baseline (see dashed line in Panel B), with substance use continuing in attempts to regain the original positive affect experienced prior to substance use. Adapted from D.J.E. Lowe et al. (ref. [16])

This also explains how substance use may be used as a form of "self-medication" in maintaining addiction, in that individuals use substances to alleviate withdrawal symptoms (see Table 8.2). Moreover, based on the dual process model of addiction,[9] an individual's automatic processes, also described as one's impulsive behavior, overshadow more executive, controlling cognition, which also maintains addictive behavior and is prominent in schizophrenia.

Substance Use in Schizophrenia and Related Disorders

Approximately half of those diagnosed with schizophrenia present a lifetime SUD.[20] Psychosis can be differentially presented, leading to a spectrum of clinical diagnoses. More chronic diagnoses, such as schizophrenia and schizoaffective disorder, are presented over a longer period of over 6 months. More acute diagnoses, such as brief psychotic disorder and schizophreniform disorder, may be present for a shorter period of time and either continue into a more chronic diagnosis or remission.[21] Moreover, substances with psychotomimetic properties, such as alcohol, cannabis, cocaine, amphetamine, and hallucinogens, can further provoke psychotic reactions and invoke a substance-induced psychosis.

Substance-induced psychosis is a psychotic episode resulting from intoxication or withdrawal of a substance. The rates of first-episode psychoses as a result of substance use in the general population range from 7% to 25%.[22] Moreover, the prevalence of substance-induced psychosis is higher among those with a mental illness. In some cases, substance-induced psychosis may transition into more chronic psychosis or classified mental disorder, such as schizophrenia, depending on the user and the substance. Certain substances have a greater risk of conversion from a substance-induced psychosis toward a chronic illness. For example, studies have found that approximately 32% of those presented with substance-induced psychosis transitioned toward bipolar or schizophrenia-spectrum disorder, with 47% of these cases as a result of cannabis use.[22] See comparison of the clinical features of substance-induced versus idiopathic (e.g., schizophrenia) psychosis in Table 8.1.

Rates of substance use are on average higher across individuals with a mental illness compared to the general population; however, substance use rates are particularly prevalent across individuals with a psychotic disorder.[23,24] There may be predisposed characteristics placing these individuals at a higher risk to substance use, such as developmental and genetic abnormalities, as well as

TABLE 8.1 ■ A Comparison of the Clinical Features of Idiopathic Versus Substance-induced Psychosis

Primary Psychosis (e.g., Schizophrenia)	Substance-Induced Psychosis
Drug urine toxicology sometimes positive	Positive substance urine toxicology
Variable reported substance use (25% prevalence of positive c urine toxicology in schizophrenia)	Heavy substance use within past month
Symptoms appear before heavy substance use	Symptoms appear only during periods of heavy substance use/sudden increase in potency
Symptoms persist despite drug abstinence	Symptoms abate or are reduced with drug abstinence
Antipsychotics markedly improve symptoms	Antipsychotics may/may not improve symptoms
Most often present with delusions, hallucinations, and thought disorder	Often associated with visual hallucinations and paranoid ideation (e.g., features of an "organic" psychosis)
Less insight about psychotic state	More aware of symptoms/insight about disease
Disorganized thought form (e.g., loose associations, tangential or circumstantial speech)	Thought form more organized and sequential

environmental and social factors that facilitate this comorbidity.[25] Regardless of the predispositions, substance use in psychotic disorders is associated with overall poorer outcomes, including higher rates of criminality, violence, hospitalization, relapse, suicide, medical comorbidities, and mortality.[1,26] Moreover, comorbid substance use has been associated with higher scores on measures of positive and negative symptoms of psychosis.[27]

Comorbid psychotic disorder and alcohol use, cigarette smoking, cannabis use, other recreational substance use (e.g., cocaine, methamphetamine, etc.), or polysubstance use is commonly observed, although research is limited and successful treatment options are lacking.[20]

ALCOHOL

Alcohol use disorder (AUD) is the most common co-occurring disorder next to nicotine in people with schizophrenia, with approximately one-third of individuals developing AUD at some point in their lives. Various studies have suggested alcohol use rates are as high as 86% in patients with schizophrenia and 65% of individuals with schizophrenia have an AUD.[20] The acute intoxication of alcohol produces greater and longer-lasting euphoria and stimulatory effects in individuals with schizophrenia.[28] These positive responses may contribute to the risk of developing AUD in this population along with alcohol's availability as a legal drug.

Although acute alcohol use induces positive feelings, it is the most common substance, next to cannabis, to induce psychosis especially in heavy, long-term alcohol users. A Finnish report found that about 4% of individuals with AUD experience alcohol-induced psychosis, and of those 95% experience varied hallucinations and 51% experience delusions.[29] Psychosis related to alcohol occurs during acute intoxication, withdrawal, and in chronic users. In most cases, alcohol-induced psychosis is dose dependent to alcohol withdrawal states, also known as alcohol withdrawal delirium. Alcohol withdrawal symptoms range from minor to severe depending on the severity of the SUD, with severe symptoms resembling a psychotic state including delirium tremens, delusions, and hallucinations that peak within a week after alcohol abstinence. More rarely, alcohol-related psychosis, or alcohol hallucinosis, presented shortly after acute intoxication, occurs in about 4% of individuals with an AUD. The symptoms include hallucinations, paranoia, and fear. Only 5% of individuals experiencing an alcohol-induced psychosis risk a schizophrenia spectrum diagnosis.[5]

Other reports have also shown the negative impact alcohol use has on physical health in patients with schizophrenia. Patients with a dual diagnosis have a twice greater chance of developing hypertension, chronic obstructive pulmonary disease, and coronary artery disease.[30] Furthermore, multiple studies have indicated the detrimental effects of alcohol on neurocognitive functioning, including impaired verbal learning, working memory, executive function, sensory gating, and higher levels of psychopathology (especially mood disturbance) and positive symptoms.[31,32]

CANNABIS

Cannabis use rates have been suggested to be as high as 80% in schizophrenia compared to the general population, and it is specifically prevalent in younger individuals and males.[20,33,34]

Delta-9-tetrahydrocannabinol (THC), a partial agonist of CB1 receptors, and cannabidiol (CBD) are the two primarily researched cannabinoids (i.e., the pharmacologic constituents of cannabis). CBD has exhibited therapeutic benefits across mental and physical disorders, while THC is psychoactive and has been correlated with psychotomimetic effects and negative implications in psychosis.[35,36]

Heavy cannabis use among the general population has been described to induce brief psychotic states, and individuals with a psychotic disorder are particularly vulnerable to relapse and aggravation of preexisting symptoms.[37] For example, among individuals with schizophrenia, comorbid cannabis use has been shown to be correlated with increased hallucinations and confusion and increased reported depression, lack of thought control, and social dysfunction.[38] This has been confirmed in clinical trials of cannabis administration in schizophrenia. For example, THC intravenously administered in individuals with schizophrenia on stable antipsychotic medication has shown to acutely heighten positive, negative, and general symptoms, as well as alter perception and worsen attention, memory, and motor stability.[35] Moreover, THC has been associated with an increased risk of psychosis in a dose-dependent manner: regular cannabis users and heavy cannabis users are two and four times more likely to develop psychosis, respectively.[39,40]

However, other reports note how individuals with schizophrenia or first-episode psychosis with a history of cannabis use have been reported to have better cognitive functioning compared to nonusers and to those who exhibited later onset of cannabis use.[41] For example, one study described how comorbid schizophrenia and cannabis use disorder were correlated with higher scores on tests of processing speed, verbal fluency, and verbal learning and memory, as well as higher scores on the global functioning scale.[42] These results have been interpreted in that cannabis use in schizophrenia may represent a higher-functioning subgroup of patients.

There is also an increased risk for earlier psychotic symptom presentation observed in conjunction with cannabis use in the general population.[43,44] Results from one of the largest longitudinal studies involving over 50,000 male participants indicate that those who smoked cannabis by the age of 18 had twice the risk for receiving a diagnosis of schizophrenia, while those who used chronically were at six times the risk compared to nonusers.[45] Notably, the administration of intravenous THC in healthy individuals has been shown to directly induce psychotic symptoms, both self-reported and assessed by the Positive and Negative Symptom Scale (PANSS).[35,46]

It has been suggested that there are different classes among those with psychotic disorders who use cannabis. One study suggests there is the group that uses to counteract the distressing symptoms of the disorder, while another group uses before the onset of the disorder, and cannabis use may have influenced presentation of symptoms.[47]

TOBACCO

Schizophrenia is known to be associated with high rates of smoking, as high as 88%, and high rates of tobacco use disorder, resulting in increased rates of morbidity and early mortality.[48] Dysregulation of nicotinic acetylcholine receptor (nAChR) systems has been proposed to increase susceptibility to smoking in schizophrenia.[25] It is thought that the high prevalence of smoking in this population is a result of genetic factors, reductions in negative symptoms when smoking, higher cravings, and remediating cognitive deficits associated with the disorder.[49] Furthermore, smoking is a common self-medication method used to ameliorate the adverse effects of antipsychotics. High-dose cigarettes have also been found to significantly decrease PANSS negative symptoms scores as well as SANS global scores[50] and have no effect on positive symptoms.

There has been no clear evidence whether tobacco use disorder may induce psychosis. It has been suggested that there is an increased risk for psychosis and earlier onset of a psychotic illness in individuals who are chronic cigarette smokers.[51] However, there needs to be more careful examination of tobacco use and first-episode psychosis.

HALLUCINOGENS

Psychedelics

Psychedelics include a variety of compounds, such as lysergic acid diethylamide (LSD), psilocybin, and mescaline, and primarily act on the serotonergic system in the brain.[52] Contrary to other substances, psychedelics have not been generally associated with long-term damage to the brain or body, nor have they been described as eliciting addictive behavior or withdrawal symptoms.[53] From a report in the United States of over 130,000 respondents, there was no correlation between psychedelic use and increased rates of mental illness, including psychosis.[52] Controlled studies have reported similar findings, with no major correlations between use and mental illness.[54] Normally, these substances induce an altered state of consciousness, with impairment in judgment posing the greatest risk for users.[55] At larger doses, however, psychotomimetic effects can be observed. For example, LSD has been described to elicit psychotic symptoms in an acute setting, similar to those observed in individuals with a psychotic disorder.[15] Psilocybin has also been shown to induce psychological consequences such as dysphoria, stress, and anxiety.[55]

Phencyclidine

Phencyclidine, also known as PCP or angel dust, is an NMDA antagonist and induces symptoms that can mirror those observed in schizophrenia.[56] Effects of use can range from altered perception, euphoria, and dysphoria to delusions and hallucinations, as well as cognitive dysfunction that individuals with schizophrenia commonly experience, which can remain prevalent even after abstinence.[56] Moreover, PCP has been used as a model of schizophrenia, as the drug commonly induces psychotic episodes, involving positive and negative symptoms, as well as cognitive disruptions.[57]

Ketamine

Ketamine is similar to psychedelics in that it is also a hallucinogenic drug, but its neurobiological action differs in the brain.[55] Ketamine is a dissociative anesthetic that has been associated with psychedelic and psychotic effects. Symptoms such as hallucinations and paranoia are commonly reported following drug administration.[58] Ketamine has been shown to induce psychotic episodes, involving positive symptom presentation, in individuals with diagnosed schizophrenia.[59] Moreover, ketamine has been shown to exacerbate existing symptoms in schizophrenia.[60] Acutely, ketamine has also been shown to induce schizophrenia-like and dissociative symptoms in healthy individuals, and has been shown to induce psychosis in healthy chronic users.[61,62]

3,4-METHYLENEDIOXY-METHAMPTHETAMINE

3,4-Methylenedioxy-methampthetamine, also known as MDMA or ecstasy, is a synthetic amphetamine that has both stimulant and hallucinogenic properties. Originally, ecstasy was used in psychotherapy for various disorders such as PTSD. Presently it is used as a recreational drug, especially among adolescents, and similarly to psychedelics, it does not have a strong addictive potential. During intoxication, ecstasy can induce intense euphoria as well as dissociative symptoms, primarily derealization, which exceed those seen in schizophrenia.[63] Although rare, chronic and high-potency doses of ecstasy may lead to an MDMA-induced psychosis that usually persists until it wears off. There have been only a handful of case reports that have shown persistent induced psychosis after single use of MDMA.[64] Research on the relationship between ecstasy and schizophrenia is scarce due to the low likelihood of ecstasy being used as a drug of abuse, especially in this population. In most cases ecstasy pills are tainted with other substances such as amphetamines and cocaine, which is more likely the cause of a persistent psychotic disorder, especially if one has a genetic predisposition to schizophrenia.

OPIOIDS

Opioids are an increasingly common problem among people with psychotic disorders, but the prevalence compared to the general population is lower. Nonetheless, because people with schizophrenia use illegal drugs like cannabis, cocaine, and methamphetamine, these illegal drugs are often tainted with illegal high-potency opioids like fentanyl, and therefore clinicians have to be aware that psychotic patients may be at risk for opioid intoxication or opioid use disorder. Thus, these patients should be screened for opioids using urine toxicology and self-report measures and should be given naloxone kits to prevent overdoses.

COCAINE

Cocaine is classified as a stimulant that influences the central nervous system, with wide-ranging effects on the brain and body.[65] More than half (up to three-fourths) of cocaine users have reported transient psychotic symptoms.[65] Cocaine has been described to induce symptoms such as paranoia, suspiciousness, and hallucinations, especially among early-onset and heavy users.[66–68] This phenomenon has been termed cocaine-induced psychosis or CIP, potentially due to heightened dopamine levels cortically and cortically in the brain caused by cocaine's blocking of dopamine uptake.[66,69] There has also been cocaine-induced psychotic disorder or CIPD, involving primarily auditory and visual hallucinations as well as paranoia, in those who experience psychotic symptoms over a greater period of time.[65]

Because of this, cocaine use has been described as particularly detrimental to the induction and course of psychotic disorders, as psychotic disorders have been linked to dysfunctional dopaminergic activity as well.[70] In a large survey of psychiatric patients, almost half of the individuals with schizophrenia presented with substance abuse behavior, while 17% of those individuals used cocaine.[24] This rate remains consistent in hospitalized patients with schizophrenia, with roughly 20% abusing cocaine.[71] Although not the most prevalent comorbidity, the deficits experienced in psychotic disorders in concurrent cocaine users is quite significant. For example, cocaine users with schizophrenia exhibit very low remission rates compared to other substances.[72] Moreover, cocaine use has been associated with further psychosocial impairments, as well as lower scores on measures of attention, memory, and problem solving.[73]

AMPHETAMINES

Methamphetamine and amphetamine are psychostimulants that have strong addictive potentials. Although similar to cocaine, amphetamines are more potent and have a longer duration of euphoria, increased energy, alertness, and libido. Drug-induced psychosis has been reported in 46% of regular users of amphetamines. Symptoms include: lack of concentration, delusions of persecution, increased motor activity, disorganization of thoughts, lack of insight, anxiety, suspicion, and auditory hallucinations.[74] Other serious adverse consequences of acute intoxication include violence and suicide.

Methamphetamine, a derivative of amphetamine, is much stronger and has quicker intoxicating effects. Individuals dependent on methamphetamine are more likely to lose their jobs, become homeless, and turn to crime. Similarly to amphetamine, prevalence of meth-induced psychotic disorder in methamphetamine users is 36.5%, with a lifetime prevalence of 42.7%.[75] Symptoms of substance-induced psychosis for methamphetamine users include affective symptoms, psychomotor agitation, and primarily positive psychotic symptoms including: auditory and visual hallucinations, persecutory delusions, ideas of reference, and disorganized speech.[76,77]

The rate of methamphetamine use disorder is 43.3% in patients with schizophrenia.[75] About 38.8% of individuals experiencing methamphetamine psychosis eventually get diagnosed with schizophrenia due to the persistent and extended psychosis that methamphetamine may cause.[78] This is seen predominately in patients who use the smoking or intravenous method of administration and have a family history of schizophrenia.[77] Long-term amphetamine users risk cognitive impairment due to reductions in striatal dopamine transporter activity, including deficits in episodic and working memory, executive functions, visuoconstruction, and psychomotor tasks.[79,80]

Clinical Features and Assessment of Substance Use Disorders in Psychosis

Many individuals struggling with schizophrenia, schizoaffective disorder, etc. have high rates of comorbidity with other SUDs. Dual-diagnosis patients are typically male, younger at illness onset, show more extrapyramidal, positive, and depressive symptoms, fewer negative symptoms, a lower quality of life, a higher incidence of violent behavior, homelessness, and unemployment as well as lower treatment compliance.[34] There are, however, certain drugs that are more likely to cause psychotic symptoms than others. These include methamphetamine, cannabis, cocaine, amphetamine, alcohol, and psychedelic and recreational drugs. Furthermore, poly-drug use may increase risk of developing psychosis and complicates treatment in individuals with a dual diagnosis.

Some early signs and symptoms of a substance-induced psychosis include, among others, isolation, poor hygiene, worsening in work or school performance, paranoia or hostility, emotional outbursts or lack of emotional expressions, and inability to concentrate or communicate. The *Diagnostic and Statistical Manual of Mental Disorder*, 5th Edition (DSM5) is a source to help clinicians diagnose patients with an SUD and psychotic-related disorders (see Table 8.2).[81] Symptoms of a SUD are withdrawal, marked tolerance, cravings, hazardous use, and social and interpersonal problems.[77]

Individuals undergoing a substance-induced psychotic disorder may present with delusions and/or hallucinations that must appear during or after specific substance intoxication or withdrawal. The psychosis also causes significant distress and impaired functioning, is not present before use of the substance, is not caused by substance-induced delirium, and last for a brief period of time. In many cases, substance-induced psychotic disorders are very similar in representation to brief psychotic disorders but can be distinguished by the fact that the cause of the psychosis was substance related and does not last for a substantial period of time after cessation. To help distinguish between the two, clinicians can conduct a urine test to determine if the cause of the psychosis is organic. In some cases, individuals may experience perceptual disturbances from intoxication or withdrawal from a drug (such as phencyclidine) that they understand to be the

TABLE 8.2 ■ The DSM-5 Diagnostic Criteria for Substance/Medication-Induced Psychotic Disorder

Substance/Medication-Induced Psychotic Disorder

A. Presence of one or both of the following symptoms:
   1. Delusions
   2. Hallucinations

B. There is evidence from the history, physical examination, or laboratory findings of both (1) and (2):
   1. The symptoms in Criterion A developed during or soon after substance intoxication or withdrawal or after exposure to a medication
   2. The involved substance/medication is capable of producing the symptoms in Criterion A

C. The disturbance is not better explained by a psychotic disorder that is not substance- or medication-induced. Such evidence of an independent psychotic disorder could include the following:
   The symptoms preceded the onset of substance/medication use; the symptoms persist for a substantial period of time (e.g., about 1 month) after the cessation of acute withdrawal or severe intoxication; or there is other evidence of an independent non-substance/medication-induced psychotic disorder (e.g., a history of recurrent non-substance/medication-related episodes)

D. The disturbance does not occur exclusively during the course of delirium

E. The disturbance causes clinically significant distress or impairment in social, occupational, or other areas of functioning

cause of the drug. If the individual has a reality that remains intact during intoxication or withdrawal, this would not be considered a substance-induced psychotic disorder.

Structured clinical interviews, self-report measures, and urine toxicology are all methods used to assess for a SUD. The Structured Clinical Interview for DSM5 (SCID-5) is a semi-structured interview that evaluates major DSM5 diagnoses, including SUDs. The most time-efficient way to assess for an SUD, especially in hospitalized patients, is to conduct a urine toxicology to screen for any substances, following a clinical assessment based on self-report measures to screen for an SUD and its severity. Some well-known clinical assessments used in SUD are the Alcohol Use Disorders Identification Test (AUDIT), the Cannabis Use Disorder Identification Test—Revised (CUDIT-R), and the Fagerström Test for Nicotine Dependence (FTND). If a SUD is detected through these measures, brief psychosocial interventions such as Motivational Interviewing (MI) have shown to motivate patients to seek treatment.

Some basic guidelines for interviewing acutely psychotic patients are included near the end of Chapter 1.

Treatment for Co-occurring Substance Use Disorders and Psychosis

Substance use in schizophrenia and related psychotic disorders makes effective treatment much more difficult to achieve. Individuals with a dual diagnosis are more likely to have low treatment compliance as well as have a longer duration of untreated psychosis.[82] It is important to differentiate between an organic or nonorganic psychosis using urine toxicology tests to determine if a substance is detected. In cases where psychosis is a result of substance abuse, the most common and effective treatment is discontinuing use and treatment with an antipsychotic drug. On the other hand, a dual diagnosis of both SUD and a related psychotic disorder requires a concomitant treatment that addresses both disorders. In the past decade, an integrative treatment approach that includes pharmacologic treatments for both the substance use and psychotic disorder along with psychosocial treatments in the same setting have been most useful and more effective when it comes to a dual diagnosis.[83]

The most effective and common pharmacologic treatment for individuals with a dual diagnosis, especially with individuals who are experiencing a substance-induced psychosis, are atypical antipsychotics. These include clozapine, olanzapine, risperidone, quetiapine, and aripiprazole. However, treatment for substance abuse varies depending on the substance. Currently, there are a limited number of pharmacologic therapies approved for SUDs (see Table 8.3). Moreover, there

TABLE 8.3 ■ **Potential Pharmacologic Treatments for Substance Use Disorders in Psychosis**

Substance Use Disorder	FDA Approved	Other
Alcohol	Disulfiram, Naltrexone (oral and injectable extended-release) and Acamprosate	Gabapentin, Topiramate
Tobacco	Varenicline, Sustained-Release Bupropion, Nicotine Replacement Therapy	rTMS
Cannabis	N/A	N-acetylcysteine
Cocaine	N/A	Bupropion, Topiramate
Opioid	Methadone, Buprenorphine, Naltrexone	N/A
Amphetamine	N/A	Naltrexone, Bupropion

rTMS, Repetitive transcranial stimulation.

are other pharmacologic treatments for concurrent disorders commonly observed in SUD, such as obsessive-compulsive disorder (OCD), melancholic depression, atypical depression, social anxiety, and panic anxiety. Proper treatment of these comorbidities may improve outcome for both SUD and psychosis. In individuals with a SUD some psychosocial interventions are very effective alongside medication. The most effective interventions for a dual diagnosis are MI, cognitive behavioral therapy (CBT), and contingency management (CM).

ALCOHOL

Treatment for AUD in schizophrenia and related psychotic disorders is particularly difficult to achieve due to high medication noncompliance in this population. An integrative treatment approach to reduce and abstain from alcohol has been shown to be most effective.

Few pharmacologic treatment trials have been conducted on individuals with AUD and comorbid schizophrenia. Presently, the most effective treatment is a combination of antipsychotics alongside medications used to treat AUD. The FDA-approved drugs effective for a reduction in alcohol use in patients with schizophrenia include disulfiram, naltrexone (oral and injectable extended-release), and acamprosate. Oral doses of naltrexone have been found to significantly reduce alcohol intake and cravings as well as significantly reduce PANSS positive, negative, and general psychopathology scores.[84] Disulfiram and acamprosate have also shown to be effective in reducing alcohol use in this population with no reports of any worsening of psychotic symptoms.[16,85] Other treatments that have shown to be efficacious in improving alcohol abstinence and improving psychotic symptoms include gabapentin and topiramate. Few trials have looked at antipsychotics or medications for AUD specifically in treatment for both disorders. Clozapine trials report that clozapine helped patients remediate psychotic symptoms as well as reduce their overall alcohol intake. Clozapine has proven to be more effective than risperidone as well as some psychosocial interventions like Alcoholics Anonymous (AA).[86] Here, too, diagnosis and treatment of comorbid disorders such as social anxiety and panic anxiety (as well as melancholic depression, atypical depression, and OCD) may improve outcome for both alcohol and psychosis.

Although medications have been very effective in reducing alcohol use, some psychosocial interventions have also been proven effective. Individuals with MI had a significant reduction in drinking days and an increase in abstinence rates when compared to subjects receiving educational treatment.[87] CM, group counseling (e.g., AA), cue exposure therapy, and relapse prevention are other treatment methods that have been proven efficacious for AUD especially when used alongside medications.

TOBACCO

There have been several treatment studies that suggest the safety and efficacy for the first-line treatments for management with schizophrenia and tobacco use. The most common treatments for tobacco use disorder in schizophrenia from most effective are varenicline, sustained-release (SR) bupropion, nicotine replacement therapy (NRT), and repetitive transcranial stimulation (rTMS).

Multiple studies have shown significant effectiveness of varenicline as a treatment for tobacco use disorder in schizophrenia. It has been shown to reduce withdrawal symptoms, smoking urges, negative affect, and subjective rewarding effects that smoking has.[88] It has also been found that varenicline improves cognition in smokers, specifically with attention and working memory, and improves positive affect.[88] SR bupropion has also been proven effective in increasing tobacco abstinence rates in schizophrenia as well as reducing negative symptoms.[89] Integrating CM or CBT into treatment with bupropion further reduces the amount of smoking in schizophrenia.[90] NRTs, which come in forms of patches, chewing gum, inhalers, nasal sprays, and lozenges, are another effective treatment for tobacco use disorder, especially when used alongside other medications. Specifically, bupropion has been proven to be well tolerated alongside NRTs (specifically high-dose patch and gum).[91]

More recently, neuromodulation has been shown to be a promising new treatment for tobacco use disorder in patients with schizophrenia. Although research is scarce, rTMS targeted at the prefrontal cortex for long periods of time has been shown to reduce tobacco use and cravings only for the short term.[92,93] Short-term high frequency of rTMS administration was found ineffective.[94] A clinical trial has also found the use of transcranial direct current stimulation (tDCS) as a way to improve cognitive deficits found in smokers, but it did not help with reductions in use and cravings.[50]

Most medications used to treat tobacco use disorder are especially effective when used alongside psychosocial interventions, primarily MI. Even one session of MI has shown to be more helpful that psychoeducational counseling and brief interventions to help individuals with schizophrenia to seek initial treatment for their tobacco use.[95] Moreover, CM, in monetary gains, significantly reduces smoking in schizophrenia, especially when used alongside bupropion.[90,96] Other interventions such as CBT, self-help methods, and cue exposure therapy may be useful.

CANNABIS

Treatment of cannabis use involves both psychotherapy and pharmacologic therapy options.[97] A range of psychotherapy models for problematic cannabis use have been tested and proven efficacious, such as aversion therapy, brief intervention therapy, CBT, voucher therapy or CM, motivational enhancement therapy, community-based therapy, and family therapy.[97,98] Longer therapies have not proven to be more advantageous compared to more brief interventions for cannabis use.[97] This has also been shown in trials for cannabis use in individuals with psychosis, in which longer intervention trials were met with high rates of relapse and did not prove more efficacious compared to the brief interventions.[99] CM has been found to enhance outcomes in, for example, CBT in individuals with cannabis use disorder.[97,100] This method of CM has also been confirmed in individuals with diagnosed schizophrenia who use cannabis, allowing for prolonged abstinence.[101]

Overall, psychotherapy interventions have not proven to be successful, therefore pharmacologic interventions have been of interest in the literature to target withdrawal, craving and abstinence. Antidepressants and anxiolytics, such as bupropion and nefazodone, cannabinoid agonists, anticonvulsants and mood stabilizers, as well as glutamatergic agents, such as N-acetylcysteine (NAC), have all been tested in cannabis use disorder.[100] NAC seems to be the most promising pharmacologic intervention for CUD thus far.[100]

COCAINE

Treatment for cocaine involves pharmacologic, psychological, and, more recently, technology-focused treatments. Classic pharmacologic agents include dopaminergic agents (such as Levodopa) and dextroamphetamine, noradrenergic agents (such as doxazosin, disulfiram, and nepicastat), GABAergic agents (including topiramate and vigabatrin), and other more novel agents (such as modafinil and the "cocaine vaccine" Therapeutic Antibodies-Cocaine Dependence (TA-CD)).[102] Antidepressants, although commonly studied in the literature, have shown the least efficacy in cocaine use disorder.[103] Bupropion, topiramate, and psychostimulants have shown low-strength efficacy, while antipsychotics have shown medium-strength efficacy.[103] With little efficacy of tested drugs and no current approved medication on the market, other interventions have been explored, including brain stimulation. A pilot study found efficacy from rTMS aimed at the dorsal lateral prefrontal cortex in individuals with cocaine use disorder.[104] Moreover, cocaine use in schizophrenia has been specifically treated with drugs including aripiprazole, risperidone, and olanzapine due to the unique dopaminergic deficit in schizophrenia leading to more prominent craving symptoms.[105–107]

Cocaine use disorder can also be treated concurrently or individually with psychotherapy treatment. Support expressive psychotherapy and cognitive therapy, for example, have shown to be improved with both group and individual drug counseling.[108] Psychosocial treatments such as MI and CBT have proven effective; however, relapse prevention and community-based efforts are additionally influential in the maintenance of abstinence.[109]

AMPHETAMINES

Although there is no established pharmacologic treatment for amphetamine use disorder, several pharmacologic treatments have been studied. Naltrexone, an opioid antagonist, has been shown to reduce amphetamine use, and bupropion has been shown to be slightly effective in reducing methamphetamine use in chronic users.[110,111] The most effective treatments for long-term use, however, are psychosocial interventions, primarily CBT and CM.[112,113]

Treatment for a dual diagnosis with amphetamine is very complex, especially since misdiagnosis for this population is very common. Many amphetamine users who also experience schizophrenia or schizoaffective disorder are misdiagnosed as having methamphetamine-induced psychosis, potentially resulting in more psychotic episodes in their lifetime. The most common medications used in amphetamine-induced psychosis are antipsychotics and benzodiazepines or neuroleptics following acute toxicity. Studies have shown that clozapine, olanzapine, haloperidol, aripiprazole, and risperidone were highly effective in reducing psychotic symptoms. Moreover, olanzapine showed greater safety and tolerability compared to haloperidol, and risperidone had greater effect on positive psychotic symptoms compared to aripiprazole.[114,115]

PSYCHEDELICS AND 3,4-METHYLENEDIOXY-METHAMPTHETAMINE

Psychedelics are not considered dependence- or addiction-inducing, and therefore there are minimal if any trials for psychotherapeutic or pharmacologic treatment.[55] If a patient has problematic use of these substances, classical psychosocial intervention would be feasible.

Similarly to psychedelics, there is no current FDA-approved treatment for MDMA abuse. Some clinical trials have reported substantial effects of duloxetine and doxazosin as a treatment for psychostimulant dependence.[116,117] Otherwise, psychosocial interventions, primarily CBT, would be most effective. Although rare, certain case reports have showed the efficacy of antipsychotics, haloperidol and olanzapine, as well as anticonvulsants, diazepam and carbamazepine, to treat an ecstasy-induced psychotic disorder.

OPIOIDS

For opioid use–dependent patients with psychosis, withdrawal management is the first step of treatment. Medically supervised withdrawal or detoxification can be conducted to manage both physical and psychological symptoms involved with opioid withdrawal, which become apparent a few days following abstinence and decline at around day 10.[118]

Methadone or buprenorphine, long-acting oral opioids, can be prescribed to relieve withdrawal symptoms that can be incrementally decreased in dose. There are also opioid-free treatments for withdrawal, such as alpha-adrenergic agonists, benzodiazepine, gut-acting opioid, naproxen (NSAID), and antiemetic, which all aid with the physical and psychological symptoms associated with withdrawal, including increased pulse rate, increased blood pressure, anxiety, insomnia, diarrhea, chills, piloerection, nausea, vomiting, and pain.[119]

Following detoxification and upon abstinence, maintenance treatment can be conducted to encourage patients to no longer use. MI, education on medication, and rewarding patients for cooperating with treatment guides, as well as self-help group involvement, are some ways to maintain abstinence.[120] Medication, such as naltrexone, methadone, and buprenorphine, can provide other maintenance therapies for those at higher risk of relapse and use following abstinence.[119]

Conclusions

While development of treatments for comorbid SUDs and psychotic disorders are in their infancy, there have been promising developments for combined medications and behavioral interventions for tobacco and alcohol in chronic psychotic patients. Moreover, when such treatment is integrated with the management of psychosis by the same clinicians in mental health settings,[83] treatment outcomes in these dually diagnosed patient are optimized.[4] However, further research on etiology and treatments in these populations is urgently needed, as impact on overall functioning and health care costs in these complex patients needs to be better addressed.

References

1. Buckley PF, Miller BJ, Lehrer DS, et al. Psychiatric comorbidities and schizophrenia. *Schizophr Bull.* 2008;35(2):383–402.
2. Winklbaur B, Ebner N, Sachs G, et al. Substance abuse in patients with schizophrenia. *Dialogues Clin Neurosci.* 2006;8(1):37.
3. Fuciec M, Mohr S, Garin C. Factors and motives associated with drop-out in an ambulatory service for patients with psychotic disorders. *Eur Psychiatry.* 2003;18(4):193–195.
4. Ziedonis DM, Smelson D, Rosenthal RN, et al. Improving the care of individuals with schizophrenia and substance use disorders: consensus recommendations. *J Psychiatr Pract.* 2005;11(5):315–339.
5. Niemi-Pynttäri JA, Sund R, Putkonen H, et al. Substance-induced psychoses converting into schizophrenia: a register-based study of 18,478 Finnish inpatient cases. *J Clin Psychiatry.* 2013;74(1):e94–e99.
6. RachBeisel J, Scott J, Dixon L. Co-occurring severe mental illness and substance use disorders: a review of recent research. *Psychiatr Serv.* 1999;50(11):1427–1434.
7. Volkow ND, Li T-K. Drug addiction: the neurobiology of behaviour gone awry. *Nat Rev Neurosci.* 2004;5(12):963.
8. Chambers RA, Krystal JH, Self DW. A neurobiological basis for substance abuse comorbidity in schizophrenia. *Biol Psychiatry.* 2001;50(2):71–83.
9. Vandermeeren R. Hebbrecht, M. The dual process model of addiction. Towards an integrated model? *Tijdschrift voor psychiatrie.* 2012;54(8):731–740.
10. Swendsen J, Conway KP, Degenhardt L, et al. Mental disorders as risk factors for substance use, abuse and dependence: results from the 10-year follow-up of the National Comorbidity Survey. *Addiction.* 2010;105(6):1117–1128.
11. Conway KP, Swendsen J, Husky MM, et al. Association of lifetime mental disorders and subsequent alcohol and illicit drug use: results from the National Comorbidity Survey–Adolescent Supplement. *J Am Acad Child Adolesc Psychiatry.* 2016;55(4):280–288.
12. Khantzian EJ. The self-medication hypothesis of substance use disorders: a reconsideration and recent applications. *Harvard Rev Psychiatry.* 1997;4(5):231–244.
13. Khantzian EJ. Reflections on treating addictive disorders: a psychodynamic perspective. *Am J Addict.* 2012;21(3):274–279.
14. Swofford CD, Scheller-Gilkey G, Miller AH, et al. Double jeopardy: schizophrenia and substance use. *Am J Drug Alcohol Abuse.* 2000;26(3):343–353.
15. Turner WM, Tsuang MT. Impact of substance abuse on the course and outcome of schizophrenia. *Schizophr Bull.* 1990;16(1):87–95.
16. Mueser KT, Noordsy DL, Fox L, et al. Disulfiram treatment for alcoholism in severe mental illness. *Am J Addict.* 2003;12(3):242–252.

17. Lowe DJE, Sasiadek JD, Coles AS, et al. Cannabis and mental illness: a review. *Eur Arch Psychiat Clin Neurosci.* 2019;269:107–120.
18. Koob GF, Le Moal M. Drug addiction, dysregulation of reward, and allostasis. *Neuropsychopharmacology.* 2001;24(2):97.
19. Wise RA, Koob GF. The development and maintenance of drug addiction. *Neuropsychopharmacology.* 2014;39(2):254.
20. Volkow ND. *Substance Use Disorders in Schizophrenia—Clinical Implications of Comorbidity.* Oxford University Press London, UK; 2009.
21. American Psychological Association. *Diagnostic and Statistical Manual of Mental Disorders.* 5th ed. Washington, DC: Author; 2013.
22. Starzer MSK, Nordentoft M, Hjorthøj C. Rates and predictors of conversion to schizophrenia or bipolar disorder following substance-induced psychosis. *Am J Psychiatry.* 2017;175(4):343–350.
23. Hartz SM, Pato CN, Medeiros H, et al. Comorbidity of severe psychotic disorders with measures of substance use. *JAMA Psychiatry.* 2014;71(3):248–254.
24. Regier DA, Farmer ME, Rae DS, et al. Comorbidity of mental disorders with alcohol and other drug abuse: results from the Epidemiologic Catchment Area (ECA) study. *JAMA.* 1990;264(19):2511–2518.
25. Kozak K, Barr MS, George TP. Traits and biomarkers for addiction risk in schizophrenia. *Curr Addiction Rep.* 2017;4(1):14–24.
26. Cantor-Graae E, Nordström L, McNeil T. Substance abuse in schizophrenia: a review of the literature and a study of correlates in Sweden. *Schizophr Res.* 2001;48(1):69–82.
27. Addy PH, Radhakrishnan R, Cortes JA, et al. Comorbid alcohol, cannabis, and cocaine use disorders in schizophrenia: epidemiology, consequences, mechanisms, and treatment. *Focus.* 2012;10(2):140–153.
28. D'Souza DC, Gil RB, Madonick S. Enhanced sensitivity to the euphoric effects of alcohol in schizophrenia. *Neuropsychopharmacology.* 2006;31(12):2767.
29. Perälä J, Kuoppasalmi K, Pirkola S, et al. Alcohol-induced psychotic disorder and delirium in the general population. *Br J Psychiatry.* 2010;197(3):200–206.
30. Batki SL, Meszaros ZS, Strutynski K, et al. Medical comorbidity in patients with schizophrenia and alcohol dependence. *Schizophr Res.* 2009;107(2–3):139–146.
31. Bowie CR, Serper MR, Riggio S, et al. Neurocognition, symptomatology, and functional skills in older alcohol-abusing schizophrenia patients. *Schizophr Bull.* 2005;31(1):175–182.
32. Manning V, Betteridge S, Wanigaratne S, et al. Cognitive impairment in dual diagnosis inpatients with schizophrenia and alcohol use disorder. *Schizophr Res.* 2009;114(1–3):98–104.
33. Koskinen J, Löhönen J, Koponen H, et al. Rate of cannabis use disorders in clinical samples of patients with schizophrenia: a meta-analysis. *Schizophr Bull.* 2009;36(6):1115–1130.
34. Barnes TR, Mutsatsa SH, Hutton SB, et al. Comorbid substance use and age at onset of schizophrenia. *Br J Psychiatry.* 2006;188(3):237–242.
35. D'Souza DC, Perry E, MacDougall L, et al. The psychotomimetic effects of intravenous delta-9-tetrahydrocannabinol in healthy individuals: implications for psychosis. *Neuropsychopharmacology.* 2004;29(8):1558.
36. Devinsky O, Cilio MR, Cross H, et al. Cannabidiol: pharmacology and potential therapeutic role in epilepsy and other neuropsychiatric disorders. *Epilepsia.* 2014;55(6):791–802.
37. Johns A. Psychiatric effects of cannabis. *Br J Psychiatry.* 2001;178(2):116–122.
38. Peters BD, de Koning P, Dingemans P, et al. Subjective effects of cannabis before the first psychotic episode. *Aust N Zeal J Psychiatry.* 2009;43(12):1155–1162.
39. Marconi A, Di Forti M, Lewis CM, et al. Meta-analysis of the association between the level of cannabis use and risk of psychosis. *Schizophr Bull.* 2016;42(5):1262–1269.
40. Di Forti M, Morgan C, Dazzan P, et al. High-potency cannabis and the risk of psychosis. *Br J Psychiatry.* 2009;195(6):488–491.
41. Yücel M, Bora E, Lubman DI, et al. The impact of cannabis use on cognitive functioning in patients with schizophrenia: a meta-analysis of existing findings and new data in a first-episode sample. *Schizophr Bull.* 2010;38(2):316–330.
42. DeRosse P, Kaplan A, Burdick KE, et al. Cannabis use disorders in schizophrenia: effects on cognition and symptoms. *Schizophr Res.* 2010;120(1–3):95–100.

43. Kelley ME, Wan CR, Broussard B, et al. Marijuana use in the immediate 5-year premorbid period is associated with increased risk of onset of schizophrenia and related psychotic disorders. *Schizophr Res.* 2016;171(1–3):62–67.
44. Helle S, Ringen PA, Melle I, et al. Cannabis use is associated with 3 years earlier onset of schizophrenia spectrum disorder in a naturalistic, multi-site sample (N = 1119). *Schizophr Res.* 2016;170(1):217–221.
45. Andréasson S, Allebeck P, Engström A, et al. Cannabis and schizophrenia a longitudinal study of swedish conscripts. *The Lancet.* 1987;330(8574):1483–1486.
46. Morrison P, Zois V, McKeown DA, et al. The acute effects of synthetic intravenous Δ9-tetrahydrocannabinol on psychosis, mood and cognitive functioning. *Psychol Med.* 2009;39(10):1607–1616.
47. Bersani G, Orlandi V, Kotzalidis GD, et al. Cannabis and schizophrenia: impact on onset, course, psychopathology and outcomes. *Eur Arch Psychiatry Clin Neurosci.* 2002;252(2):86–92.
48. Ziedonis DM, Hitsman B, Beckham JC, et al. *Tobacco Use and Cessation in Psychiatric Disorders. National Institutes of Mental Health Report. Nicotine Tob. Res.* 2008;10:1691–1715.
49. Lucatch AM, Lowe DJE, Clark RC, et al. Neurobiological determinants of tobacco smoking in schizophrenia. *Front in Psychiatry.* 2018;9:672.
50. Smith RC, Boules S, Mattiuz S, et al. Effects of transcranial direct current stimulation (tDCS) on cognition, symptoms, and smoking in schizophrenia: a randomized controlled study. *Schizophr Res.* 2015;168(1–2):260–266.
51. Gurillo P, Jauhar S, Murray RM, et al. Does tobacco use cause psychosis? Systematic review and meta-analysis. *Lancet Psychiatry.* 2015;2(8):718–725.
52. Krebs TS, Johansen P-Ø. Psychedelics and mental health: a population study. *PLoS One.* 2013;8(8):e63972.
53. Nichols DE. Hallucinogens. *Pharmacol Therapeutics.* 2004;101(2):131–181.
54. Studerus E, Kometer M, Hasler F, et al. Acute, subacute and long-term subjective effects of psilocybin in healthy humans: a pooled analysis of experimental studies. *J Psychopharmacol.* 2011;25(11):1434–1452.
55. Nichols DE. Psychedelics. *Pharmacol Rev.* 2016;68(2):264–355.
56. Murray JB. Phencyclidine (PCP): a dangerous drug, but useful in schizophrenia research. *J Psychol.* 2002;136(3):319–327.
57. Javitt DC, Zukin SR. Recent advances in the phencyclidine model of schizophrenia. *Am J Psychiatry.* 1991;148(10):1301–1308.
58. Lim D. Ketamine associated psychedelic effects and dependence. *Singapore Med J.* 2003;44(1):31–34.
59. Lahti AC, Koffel B, LaPorte D, et al. Subanesthetic doses of ketamine stimulate psychosis in schizophrenia. *Neuropsychopharmacology.* 1995;13(1):9–19.
60. Malhotra AK, Pinals DA, Adler CM, et al. Ketamine-induced exacerbation of psychotic symptoms and cognitive impairment in neuroleptic-free schizophrenics. *Neuropsychopharmacology.* 1997;17(3):141.
61. Morgan CJ, Mofeez A, Brandner B, et al. Acute effects of ketamine on memory systems and psychotic symptoms in healthy volunteers. *Neuropsychopharmacology.* 2004;29(1):208.
62. Morgan CJ, Curran HV. Independent Scientific Committee on Drugs. Ketamine use: a review. *Addiction.* 2012;107(1):27–38.
63. van Heugten-Van der Kloet D, Giesbrecht T, van Wel J, et al. MDMA, cannabis, and cocaine produce acute dissociative symptoms. *Psychiatry Res.* 2015;228(3):907–912.
64. Patel A, Moreland T, Haq F, et al. Persistent psychosis after a single ingestion of "Ecstasy" (MDMA). *Primary Care Comp CNS Disord.* 2011;13(6). PCC.11l01200.
65. Tang Y, Martin NL, Cotes RO. Cocaine-induced psychotic disorders: presentation, mechanism, and management. *J Dual Diagn.* 2014;10(2):98–106.
66. Roncero C, Daigre C, Gonzalvo B, et al. Risk factors for cocaine-induced psychosis in cocaine-dependent patients. *Eur Psychiatry.* 2013;28(3):141–146.
67. Floyd AG, Boutros NN, Struve FA, et al. Risk factors for experiencing psychosis during cocaine use: a preliminary report. *J Psychiatr Res.* 2006;40(2):178–182.
68. Vorspan F, Bloch V, Brousse G, et al. Prospective assessment of transient cocaine-induced psychotic symptoms in a clinical setting. *Am J Addict.* 2011;20(6):535–537.
69. Smith MJ, Thirthalli J, Abdallah AB, et al. Prevalence of psychotic symptoms in substance users: a comparison across substances. *Compr Psychiatry.* 2009;50(3):245–250.
70. Meltzer HY, Stahl SM. The dopamine hypothesis of schizophrenia: a review. *Schizophr Bull.* 1976;2(1):19.

71. Shaner A, Khalsa ME, Roberts L, et al. Unrecognized cocaine use among schizophrenic patients. *Am J Psychiatry*. 1993;150(5):758–762.
72. Bell M, Greig T, Gill P, et al. Work rehabilitation and patterns of substance use among persons with schizophrenia. *Psychiatr Serv*. 2002;53(1):63–69.
73. O'Malley S, Adamse M, Heaton RK, et al. Neuropsychological impairment in chronic cocaine abusers. *Am J Drug Alcohol Abuse*. 1992;18(2):131–144.
74. Bramness JG, Gundersen ØH, Guterstam J, et al. Amphetamine-induced psychosis—a separate diagnostic entity or primary psychosis triggered in the vulnerable? *BMC Psychiatry*. 2012;12(1):221.
75. Lecomte T, Dumais A, Dugré JR, et al. The prevalence of substance-induced psychotic disorder in methamphetamine misusers: a meta-analysis. *Psychiatry Res*. 2018;268:189–192.
76. Wearne TA, Cornish JL. A comparison of methamphetamine-induced psychosis and schizophrenia: a review of positive, negative, and cognitive symptomatology. *Front Psychiatry*. 2018;9:491.
77. McKetin R, Dawe S, Burns RA, et al. The profile of psychiatric symptoms exacerbated by methamphetamine use. *Drug Alcohol Depend*. 2016;161:104–109.
78. Kittirattanapaiboon P, Mahatnirunkul S, Booncharoen H, et al. Long-term outcomes in methamphetamine psychosis patients after first hospitalisation. *Drug Alcohol Rev*. 2010;29(4):456–461.
79. Volkow ND, Chang L, Wang G-J, et al. Association of dopamine transporter reduction with psychomotor impairment in methamphetamine abusers. *Am J Psychiatry*. 2001;158(3):377–382.
80. Scott JC, Woods SP, Matt GE, et al. Neurocognitive effects of methamphetamine: a critical review and meta-analysis. *Neuropsychol Rev*. 2007;17(3):275–297.
81. American Psychiatric Association. *Diagnostic and Statistical Manual of Mental Disorders*. 5th ed. Arlington, VA: American Psychiatric Association.
82. Green AI, Tohen MF, Hamer RM, et al. First episode schizophrenia-related psychosis and substance use disorders: acute response to olanzapine and haloperidol. *Schizophr Res*. 2004;66(2–3):125–135.
83. Drake R, Mercer-McFadden C, Mueser KT, et al. Review of integrated mental health and substance abuse treatment for patients with dual disorders. *Schizophr Bull*. 1998;24(4):589–608.
84. Batki SL, Dimmock JA, Wade M, et al. Monitored naltrexone without counseling for alcohol abuse/dependence in schizophrenia-spectrum disorders. *Am J Addict*. 2007;16(4):253–259.
85. Ralevski E, O'Brien E, Jane JS, et al. Treatment with acamprosate in patients with schizophrenia spectrum disorders and comorbid alcohol dependence. *J Dual Diagn*. 2011;7(1–2):64–73.
86. Drake RE, Xie H, McHugo GJ, et al. The effects of clozapine on alcohol and drug use disorders among patients with schizophrenia. *Schizophr Bull*. 2000;26(2):441–449.
87. Graeber DA, Moyers TB, Griffith G, et al. A pilot study comparing motivational interviewing and an educational intervention in patients with schizophrenia and alcohol use disorders. *Community Ment Health J*. 2003;39(3):189–202.
88. Patterson F, Jepson C, Strasser AA, et al. Varenicline improves mood and cognition during smoking abstinence. *Biol Psychiatry*. 2009;65(2):144–149.
89. George TP, Vessicchio JC, Termine A, et al. A placebo controlled trial of bupropion for smoking cessation in schizophrenia. *Biol Psychiatry*. 2002;52(1):53–61.
90. Tidey JW, Rohsenow DJ, Kaplan GB, et al. Effects of contingency management and bupropion on cigarette smoking in smokers with schizophrenia. *Psychopharmacology*. 2011;217(2):279–287.
91. George TP, Vessicchio JC, Sacco KA, et al. A placebo-controlled trial of bupropion combined with nicotine patch for smoking cessation in schizophrenia. *Biol Psychiatry*. 2008;63(11):1092–1096.
92. Amiaz R, Levy D, Vainiger D, et al. Repeated high-frequency transcranial magnetic stimulation over the dorsolateral prefrontal cortex reduces cigarette craving and consumption. *Addiction*. 2009;104(4):653–660.
93. Prikryl R, Ustohal L, Kucerova HP, et al. Repetitive transcranial magnetic stimulation reduces cigarette consumption in schizophrenia patients. *Progr Neuro Psychopharmacol Biol Psychiatry*. 2014;49:30–35.
94. Kozak K, Sharif-Razi M, Morozova M, et al. Effects of short-term, high-frequency repetitive transcranial magnetic stimulation to bilateral dorsolateral prefrontal cortex on smoking behavior and cognition in patients with schizophrenia and non-psychiatric controls. *Schizophr Res*. 2018;197:441–443.
95. Steinberg ML, Ziedonis DM, Krejci JA, et al. Motivational interviewing with personalized feedback: a brief intervention for motivating smokers with schizophrenia to seek treatment for tobacco dependence. *J Consult Clin Psychol*. 2004;72(4):723.

96. Tidey JW, O'Neill SC, Higgins ST. Contingent monetary reinforcement of smoking reductions, with and without transdermal nicotine, in outpatients with schizophrenia. *Exp Clin Psychopharmacol.* 2002;10(3):241.

97. Nordstrom BR, Levin FR. Treatment of cannabis use disorders: a review of the literature. *Am J Addict.* 2007;16(5):331–342.

98. Copeland J, Swift W. Cannabis use disorder: epidemiology and management. *Int Rev Psychiatry.* 2009;21(2):96–103.

99. Baker AL, Hides L, Lubman DI. Treatment of cannabis use among people with psychotic or depressive disorder: a systematic review. *J Clin Psychiatry.* 2010;71(3):247–254.

100. Sherman BJ, McRae-Clark AL. Treatment of cannabis use disorder: current science and future outlook. *Pharmacother J Hum Pharmacol Drug Ther.* 2016;36(5):511–535.

101. Rabin RA, Kozak K, Zakzanis KK, et al. A method to achieve extended cannabis abstinence in cannabis dependent patients with schizophrenia and non-psychiatric controls. *Schizophr Res.* 2018;194:47–54.

102. Shorter D, Domingo CB, Kosten TR. Emerging drugs for the treatment of cocaine use disorder: a review of neurobiological targets and pharmacotherapy. *Exp Opin Emerg Drugs.* 2015;20(1):15–29.

103. Chan B, Kondo K, Freeman M, et al. Pharmacotherapy for cocaine use disorder—a systematic review and meta-analysis. *J Gen Intern Med.* 2019;34(12):2858–2873.

104. Terraneo A, Leggio L, Saladini M, et al. Transcranial magnetic stimulation of dorsolateral prefrontal cortex reduces cocaine use: a pilot study. *Eur Neuropsychopharmacol.* 2016;26(1):37–44.

105. Tsuang JW, Eckman T, Marder S, et al. Can risperidone reduce cocaine use in substance abusing schizophrenic patients? *J Clin Psychopharmacol.* 2002;22(6):629–630.

106. Beresford TP, Clapp L, Martin B, et al. Aripiprazole in schizophrenia with cocaine dependence: a pilot study. *J Clin Psychopharmacol.* 2005;25(4):363–366.

107. Green AI. Pharmacotherapy for schizophrenia and co-occurring substance use disorders. *Neurotoxicity Res.* 2007;11(1):33–39.

108. Crits-Christoph P, Siqueland L, Blaine J, et al. Psychosocial treatments for cocaine dependence: National Institute on Drug Abuse collaborative cocaine treatment study. *Arch Gen Psychiatry.* 1999;56(6):493–502.

109. Carroll KM. Relapse prevention as a psychosocial treatment: a review of controlled clinical trials. *Exp Clin Psychopharmacol.* 1996;4(1):46.

110. Jayaram-Lindström N, Hammarberg A, Beck O, et al. Naltrexone for the treatment of amphetamine dependence: a randomized, placebo-controlled trial. *Am J Psychiatry.* 2008;165(11):1442–1448.

111. McCann DJ, Li SH. A novel, nonbinary evaluation of success and failure reveals bupropion efficacy versus methamphetamine dependence: reanalysis of a multisite trial. *CNS Neurosci Ther.* 2012;18(5):414–418.

112. Smout MF, Longo M, Harrison S, et al. Psychosocial treatment for methamphetamine use disorders: a preliminary randomized controlled trial of cognitive behavior therapy and acceptance and commitment therapy. *Subst Abuse.* 2010;31(2):98–107.

113. Rawson RA, McCann MJ, Flammino F, et al. A comparison of contingency management and cognitive-behavioral approaches for stimulant-dependent individuals. *Addiction.* 2006;101(2):267–274.

114. Leelahanaj T, Kongsakon R, Netrakom P. A 4-week, double-blind comparison of olanzapine with haloperidol in the treatment of amphetamine psychosis. *J Med Assoc Thailand= Chotmaihet thangphaet.* 2005;88:S43–S52.

115. Farnia V, Shakeri J, Tatari F, et al. Randomized controlled trial of aripiprazole versus risperidone for the treatment of amphetamine-induced psychosis. *Am J Drug Alcohol Abuse.* 2014;40(1):10–15.

116. Hysek CM, Simmler LD, Nicola VG, et al. Duloxetine inhibits effects of MDMA ("Ecstasy") in vitro and in humans in a randomized Placebo-Controlled Laboratory Study. *PLoS One.* 2012;7(5):e36476.

117. Hysek CM, Fink AE, Simmler LD, et al. α1-adrenergic receptors contribute to the acute effects of 3,4-methylenedioxymethamphetamine in humans. *J Clin Psychopharmacol.* 2013;33(5):658–666.

118. Sigmon SC, Bisaga A, Nunes EV, et al. Opioid detoxification and naltrexone induction strategies: recommendations for clinical practice. *Am J Drug Alcohol Abuse.* 2012;38(3):187–199.

119. Schuckit MA. Treatment of opioid-use disorders. *N Engl J Med.* 2016;375(4):357–368.

120. Dutra L, Stathopoulou G, Basden SL, et al. A meta-analytic review of psychosocial interventions for substance use disorders. *Am J Psychiatry.* 2008;165(2):179–187.

CHAPTER 9

Psychoses Due to Medical Illness or Iatrogenesis

Gilberto Sousa Alves ■ Leandro Oliveira Trovão ■ Lucas Briand

Abstract

Medical illness–related and medical treatment–related (iatrogenic) psychoses are caused by the direct effects of a medical condition or treatment-related medications or other interventions. Prevalence varies by age, genetic and familial characteristics, previous history of psychiatric problems, environmental exposure to chemical agents, pesticides, access to medication, and medical comorbidities (e.g., hypothyroidism). These psychoses are more commonly due to medications or drugs among young adults, while elderly patients more commonly have structural brain changes and dementia. Since a wide range of potential etiologies are possible, diagnostic evaluation starts with extensive clinical history and physical examination, as well as serologic, biological, and neuroimaging procedures. In this chapter, the most important causes of medical illness and medical treatment–induced psychotic disorders are described and discussed, including diagnostic classification, symptomatology, and treatment.

KEYWORDS

Psychosis and organic
Psychosis and herpes
Organic psychosis and dementia

Secondary psychosis
Psychosis and syphilis
Alzheimer and psychosis

Psychosis and dementia
Organic psychosis
Organic psychosis and causes

Introduction

Psychotic disorders are clinical conditions characterized by major changes in thought and critical judgment, affecting individual relationships while also impairing functioning and quality. Unlike primary psychiatric conditions, where etiology is thought to be an interaction between genetic vulnerability and exposure to stressors, in organic psychoses a medical condition or treatment underlies the behavioral changes and typically determines treatment, outcome, and prognosis. In the *Diagnostic and Statistical Manual of Mental Disorders*, 5th Edition (DSM-5; Tables 9.1 and 9.2), organic psychosis can be classified in the topics substance/medication-induced psychotic disorder and psychotic disorder due to another medical condition.[1] (See Fig. 9.1.)

In most cases, the evolution of organic psychosis varies from ordinary psychotic disorders, which more often have high rates of family abandonment, other psychiatric comorbidities, social and marital impairment, and work problems. The spectrum of clinical conditions potentially relating to the occurrence of psychotic disturbances is extremely broad and includes infectious, autoimmune, inflammatory, neurodegenerative, metabolic, and cardiovascular mechanisms (Tables 9.3 and 9.4).

TABLE 9.1 ■ DSM-5 Diagnostic Criteria (American Psychiatry Association) for Substance/Medication-Induced Psychosis

(1) Substance/medication-induced psychotic disorder — diagnostic criteria

A. Presence of one or both of the following symptoms:
   1. Delusions.
   2. Hallucinations.

B. There is evidence from the history, physical examination, or laboratory findings of both (1) and (2):
   1. **The symptoms in Criterion A developed during or soon after substance intoxication or withdrawal or after exposure to a medication.**
   2. **The involved substance/medication is capable of producing the symptoms in Criterion A.**

C. The disturbance is not better explained by a psychotic disorder that is not substance/medication-induced. Such evidence of an independent psychotic disorder could include the following:
   The symptoms preceded the onset of the substance/medication use; the symptoms persist for a **substantial period of time (e.g., about 1 month) after the cessation of acute withdrawal or severe intoxication; or there is other evidence of an independent non-substance/medication-induced psychotic disorder (e.g., a history of recurrent non-substance/medication-related episodes).**

D. The disturbance does not occur exclusively during the course of a delirium.

E. The disturbance causes clinically significant distress or impairment in social, occupational, or other important areas of functioning.

Note: This diagnosis should be made instead of a diagnosis of substance intoxication or substance withdrawal only when the symptoms in Criterion A predominate in the clinical picture and when sufficiently severe to deserve clinical attention.

From Substance/Medication-Induced Psychotic Disorder, American Psychiatric Association. Schizophrenia spectrum and other psychotic disorders. In: *Diagnostic and Statistical Manual of Mental Disorders*. 5th ed. 2013:110. https://doi.org/10.1176/appi.books.9780890425596.dsm02.

TABLE 9.2 ■ DSM-5 Diagnostic Criteria 293.8x (F06.x) (American Psychiatry Association) for Illness-related Psychosis

(2) Psychotic disorder due to another medical condition — diagnostic criteria

A. Prominent hallucinations or delusions.

B. There is evidence from the history, physical examination, or laboratory findings that the disturbance is the direct pathophysiologic consequence of another medical condition.

C. The disturbance is not better explained by another mental disorder.

D. The disturbance does not occur exclusively during the course of a delirium.

E. The disturbance causes clinically significant distress or impairment in social, occupational, or other important areas of functioning.

From Psychotic Disorder Due to Another Medical Condition & American Psychiatric Association. Schizophrenia spectrum and other psychotic disorders. In: *Diagnostic and Statistical Manual of Mental Disorders*. 5th ed. 2013:115 — code 293. 8x, F06.x. https://doi.org/10.1176/appi.books.9780890425596.dsm02.

Medication-induced psychosis is commonly related to certain specific drug categories and treatment regimens. Iatrogenic psychoses can have severe outcomes, including new-onset or worsened chronic disability, and can render clinical management extraordinarily difficult.[2] In certain cases, psychosis precedes more severe and overt toxicity, which can lead to encephalopathy and central nervous system (CNS) depression.

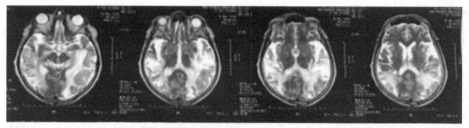

Fig. 9.1 T2 images (axial slices) showing large involvement of the bilateral parietal and occipital regions, as well as temporal impairment in one patient with herpetic encephalitis.

TABLE 9.3 ■ **Main Etiologies of Medical Illness-related Psychosis**

Dementia and other neurodegenerative causes of psychosis	
• Alzheimer disease	• Pick disease
• Vascular dementia	• Huntington disease
• Parkinson disease and Lewy body dementia	• Creutzfeldt-Jakob Disease

TABLE 9.4 ■ **Main Etiologies of Medical Illness-related Psychosis**

Medical illness-related psychosis: causes	
• Dementia and other neurodegenerative diseases	• Nutritional
• Infections	• Prions
• Autoimmune	• Paraneoplastic syndromes
• Endocrine-metabolic	• Substance/drug abuse or use
• Dementia and other neurodegenerative diseases	• Nutritional

In this chapter, the most important causes of organic psychotic disorders, their diagnosis, symptoms, and treatment are described and discussed.

Neurobiology and Putative Mechanisms of Organic Psychosis

The increasing knowledge of neurobiology in mental disorders has enabled further understanding of the relationship between changes in brain structure to functional and psychotic manifestations.

GENETIC AND NEUROIMAGING STUDIES

Genetic studies on first-episode psychosis have investigated the role of auto-antibodies associated with encephalitis in the autoimmune encephalitis with anti-N-methyl-D-aspartate (NMDA) and encephalopathy associated with autoimmune thyroid diseases (EAATDs).[3] Putative mechanisms relating NMDA receptors to psychosis comprise down-regulation of glutamate receptors. The most frequent genetic syndrome implicated in schizophrenia is 22q11.2 deletion syndrome (DS), whose incidence is estimated in the range of 4300 to 7000 live births.[4] Four classical chromosomal anomalies leading to psychosis include Prader-Willi syndrome, Turner syndrome, Klinefelter syndrome, and juvenile-onset Huntington disease, defined as onset before age 20, seen in 5% of cases.[3] Table 9.2: DSM-5 diagnostic criteria (American Psychiatry Association) in psychosis due to a medical condition.

Several brain regions have been implicated in the pathophysiology of psychotic-related symptoms, for instance the temporal, ventromedial, and orbitofrontal cortex, the anterior cingulate, and the *nucleus accumbens*.[5-8] In addition, behavior disturbances may result from neuronal disruption in specific networks; as a matter of example, the cholinergic transmission might be affected by a disruption in the anterior cingulate, insula, lateral frontal, and lateral temporal circuits, leading to agitation and aggression.[9] In patients with age-related cognitive disorders, including Alzheimer disease (AD) and mild cognitive impairment, the occurrence of psychosis[10-16] and agitation[10,14,17-19] is regarded as among the most common features during disease progression. Most of these patients also present aberrant motor activity,[20,21] delusions,[22] and hallucinations.[23]

More recent neuroimaging techniques are able to explore the neuroradiologic underpinnings of organic psychosis. Using single-photon emission computed tomography (SPECT), organic psychotic symptoms have been associated with lower perfusion in distinct areas, including the prefrontal cortex (bilaterally), the left anterior cingulate, ventral striatum and pulvinar areas,[13] the parietal lobe,[10,13] and the right occipital lobe.[10]

Some of these findings are similar to neuroanatomical abnormalities prodromally noted in functional psychosis patients. In particular, prefrontal cortex dysfunction may predispose to various psychoses (see Chapter 2). Paranoid symptoms have also been related to cortical thinning in the left medial orbitofrontal and superior temporal areas,[16] and delusion and hallucination were also associated with vascular lacunae in the left basal ganglia.[14] In one SPECT study,[20] the severity of symptoms was associated with lower regional cerebral flow in parietal-temporal lobes in the AD group. These findings suggest that major pathologic events compromising brain-distributed networks, particularly those involved in the emotional regulation, inhibition and reward control, and sensorial interpretation (i.e., visual and auditory stimulus), underlie some of the psychopathologic features commonly reported in AD.

Neuronal networks from the right hemisphere are thought to regulate social and sexual behavior.[24] Agitated behavior in AD seems to have a right hemisphere predominance.[10] In addition, the temporal and inferior frontal lobes[10] and the basal ganglia[14] might also participate in emotional regulation, as demonstrated by studies with AD. Indeed, previous histopathologic evidence has indicated that poorer social judgment and inappropriateness of behavior in AD may be associated with neurofibrillary tangles in the orbitofrontal cortex.[10,25]

Seizure-related psychosis usually involves frontal and mesial temporal dysfunction. According to Bear and colleagues,[26,27] temporal lobe epilepsy (TLE) may result from altered regulation and increased connectivity of sensory limbic circuitry, mostly as a result of progressive changes secondary to epilepsy activity in these areas, clinically acknowledged as the *kindling effect*. Other findings related to epilepsy also include inter-hemisphere asymmetry, including smaller right temporal volume and reduced positron emission tomography (PET) metabolism in frontal, basal ganglia, and temporal areas.[28]

Interestingly, psychosis-related changes were often reported in the anterior portion of the brain. In age-related disorders, these changes could also be found in mild cognitive impairment subjects and included higher atrophy in frontal[12,15] and parietal areas,[12] cingulate,[22] anterior cingulate, and fornix.[29] Conversely, age-related brain changes are often associated with cognitive decline and decrease in cognitive reserve, representing one major risk factor for drug- or medication-induced psychosis, particularly among the elderly.

Epidemiology

The prevalence of medical illness–related psychosis in the different age groups correlates directly with the underlying cause, that is, the related etiologic agent, as well as with varied sociodemographic characteristics. For example, these include exposure to bacterial and viral infectious pathogens, positive family history of autoimmune diseases, and socioeconomic characteristics (adequate nutrition conditions, basic health service access, vaccinations, regular pediatric visits). Occupational factors include exposure to neurotoxic pathogens such as mercury and lead among beauticians, painters, pesticide handlers, farmers, and mine workers. Duration of exposure and the absorbed dose are relevant prognostic factors. In adults, the use of licit and illicit drugs, such as cocaine, marijuana, and synthetic drugs, can trigger changes in thinking, such as paranoid ideation, as well as agitation and restlessness (see Chapter 8). The occurrence of psychosis in users of amphetamine may reach 100% and 80% in the case of cannabis and cocaine, respectively.[30] Such changes can be identified in acute or chronic intoxication and in abstinence.

Approximately 80% of patients with systemic *lupus erythematosus* (SLE) develop psychotic symptoms within the first year of diagnosis[31] and of these, 5.4% seem to present medication-induced psychosis.[32] As already outlined, the aging process also greatly increases the occurrence of organic psychotic phenomena.[33] Factors that are classically linked to aging, such as increased occurrence of heart disease (including atrial fibrillation and other arrhythmias), peripheral and cerebral vascular disease, regional volumetric changes of degenerative origin in the limbic system as well as temporal and frontal area structures, may each be determinants. Paraneoplastic manifestations and neurologic tumors should also be considered, especially if endocrine or CNS.

Classification of Medical Illness-Related Psychosis

A large number of potential conditions leading to psychotic disturbances should be considered (see Tables 9.3 and 9.4). They often vary according to age range, genetic and familiar characteristics, previous history of behavior disturbance, environmental exposure to chemical agents, pesticides, access to medication, and medical comorbidities. Thus, medical causes of psychosis can derive from multiple potential clinical causes, for example, dementia, metabolic disorders (e.g., hypothyroidism, Wilson disease, Niemann-Pick type C, porphyria), medications, or use or abuse of substances. Establishing underlying organic diagnoses is essential to determining proper treatment and prognosis.

DEGENERATIVE AND OTHER NEUROLOGIC CAUSES

One of the leading causes of medical illness-related psychosis is aging-related disorders. An estimated 40% to 60% of AD patients, for instance, experience hallucinations and delusions. The presence of psychotic symptoms in dementia increases the deterioration of life quality and accelerates institutionalization.[34] In Lewy body dementia (LBD), visual hallucinations are one hallmark of the disease. Psychosis can be seen also in frontotemporal dementia (FTD), Pick disease, and Huntington disease. Behavior disturbances seem to be closely related to regional brain atrophy and specific network disconnection, rather than resulting from global brain degeneration. Inappropriate behaviors, like agitation, may be the result of inadequate activation of the salient network, in areas such as the insula,[18] amygdala,[18] striatum, and anterior cingulate.

Parkinson's disease (PD) affects 1 in 100 individuals over 60,[35] with new cases increasing in advanced age groups, reaching a 14% incidence rate above 70 years. Psychotic symptoms usually occur secondary to pharmacologic treatment with levodopa and dopamine agonist agents.

The basic distinction between PD and LBD would be the early occurrence of cognitive symptoms in the latter, while in PD, motor symptoms usually precede cognitive deterioration. The occurrence of dementia in PD may be linked to such predictive factors as delusions and visual or auditory hallucinations. About 61% of patients with PD exhibit neuropsychiatric disorders, with hallucinations present in 27% of cases.[36] Symptoms such as advanced age, history of depression, and sleep disorder are also considered predictors of psychosis.

Vascular dementia, secondary to stroke, can present with psychotic features, especially when the lesion is in the right temporo-parieto-occipital area. Other areas of the brain are also associated with hallucinations when injured by stroke. The occurrence of psychosis in vascular disease can reach 46%.[37] The occurrence of psychosis may be related to decreased perfusion in the parietal lobe left anterior cingulate and prefrontal cortex.[33]

Psychosis of epilepsy usually encompasses a wide group of disorders with etiopathogenetic mechanisms believed to be directly connected to seizure disorder. The prevalence of such conditions may be considerably higher than primary forms of schizophrenia, ranging from 7% to 10%. Most clinical manifestations, around 25% of cases, occur in post-ictal states, where the occurrence of confusion or psychotic features follows 1 week or less after a seizure.

NUTRITIONAL CAUSES

Pellagra, a chronic niacin (vitamin B3) deficiency, usually relates to malnutrition or chronic exposure to alcohol. Niacin is contained in such common foods as grains, cereals, meat, peanuts, eggs, and fish, so pellagra incidence is declining in the general population. Classic clinical manifestations comprise the triad of dermatitis, dementia, and diarrhea. The *dementia component* of pellagra includes not only cognitive deficits but also a range of neuropsychiatric disorders such as confusion, affective disorders, and psychotic symptoms.

Vitamin B12 deficiency is a common condition, related to megaloblastic anemia and neurologic and psychiatric disorders. Among the psychiatric disorders described, a psychotic disorder secondary to vitamin B12 deficiency is possible, though uncommon. Neuropsychiatric disorders may occur concomitantly with anemia or even in their absence, making this diagnosis quite difficult to establish. It is important to investigate the cause of the patient's deficiency, whether it is due to medication use (e.g., metformin), low dietary intake of B12, pernicious anemia, or other conditions.

NEUROTOXIC CAUSES

Neuropsychiatric disorders associated with occupational exposure to substances such as cosmetics, paints, and pesticides are noted above. Exposure to zinc has been linked to the development of depression, anxiety, and psychosis in animal models. Exposure to lead, which is mainly related to leaded paint, can lead to a state similar to porphyria, with such neuropsychiatric changes as delusions and hallucinations, along with neurologic changes such as weakness. Pesticides, besides being important risk factors for the development of cancers and teratogenicity, may also contribute to neuropsychiatric disorders, primarily to the development of dementias such as AD and PD.

INFECTIOUS CAUSES

Bacterial, virus, or fungi infections of CNS are often associated with organic psychosis. Herpes simplex encephalitis, caused especially by herpes simplex virus type 1, is a rare presentation of the herpes simplex infection. The clinical presentation is often fever associated with neurologic symptoms, but neuropsychiatric symptoms, such as psychotic symptoms, may occur. Diagnosis is made by biochemical abnormalities and Polymerase chain reaction (PCR) positive for herpes simplex virus in the cerebral-spinal fluid. Tertiary syphilis may rarely present with psychosis. Major symptoms usually include ataxia, headache, dizziness, and pupillary changes (i.e., Argyll-Robertson reflex). Diagnosis can be made by a Venereal Disease Research Laboratory (VDRL)-reactive test in the cerebral spinal fluid.

Psychosis secondary to arboviruses is another rare condition. Cases involving infection transmitted by the Aedes mosquitoes, such as dengue virus, Chikungunya, or Zika, and usually manifested with self-limited exanthematic disease, were reported as followed by psychotic manifestations and neurologic complications in South America[38] and Asia.[39]

Although infrequent, psychotic findings due to severe tuberculosis may occur, particularly when the microbe reaches the Substantia nigra (dopamine synthesis center). Neurologic changes usually follow tuberculous meningitis and are more likely to occur among immune-compromised individuals. The clinical presentation also includes fever, headache, and neck stiffness. Neuropsychiatric disorders, including psychosis, may occur at the onset or further along the disease course. Such microbes as *Borrelia*, *Mycoplasma*, and *Chlamydia*, among others, may cause neuropsychiatric symptoms due to CNS infection.

OTHER INFECTIOUS AGENTS

Other tropical diseases encompass psychotic manifestations and CNS complications as major clinical presentations. In neurocysticercosis, behavior changes, including psychotic symptoms, have been reported.[40] These symptoms may occur due to structural damage to the brain parenchyma caused by the disease itself, or as a side effect of its treatment. In malaria, especially when there is encephalic involvement, neuropsychiatric manifestations may occur, among them psychosis. Diseases caused by protozoa of the Trypanosomatidae family, such as Chagas disease *(Trypanosoma cruzi)* and sleeping sickness *(Trypanosoma brucei gambiense)*, may also have psychiatric involvement. In the former, although encephalic involvement has been demonstrated, clinical neurologic manifestations are rare and generally transient. In sleeping sickness, hypersomnia may be accompanied by paranoia, hallucinations, and delusions. In Creutzfeldt-Jakob-Disease, a prionic disease, psychotic symptoms can accompany neurologic symptoms such as dementia, tremor, and language disturbances.

ENDOCRINE-METABOLIC CAUSES

Thyroid disease is commonly associated with behavior disturbances, regardless of its etiology. Clinical manifestation of *hypo*-thyroidism is commonly associated with irritability, anxiety, and mood symptoms, particularly depression. Hashimoto's thyroiditis is a common cause of *hypo*-throidism, and can also lead to Hashimoto's encephalopathy. The occurrence of psychotic crisis due to *hyper*-thyroidism or thyroid storm, is unusual, although psychotic symptoms associated with the rapid correction of high levels of fT4 to hypothyroidism in the form of "myxedema madness" are well described.[41] Psychotic symptoms due to thyroid dysfunction may be accompanied by atypical features, including catatonia, multiple-modality hallucinations, and elevated anti-thyroglobulin and anti-Thyroid peroxidase (TPO) antibodies.[41]

GENETIC CAUSES

Wilson's disease is an autosomal recessive disease of copper metabolism, usually manifested between 6 and 60 years, most commonly affecting individuals in the first two decades of life. The dysfunction is caused by a change in the copper P-ATPase transporting enzyme and causes a disturbance in copper excretion and deposition,[42] later affecting the kidneys and corneas. There are several mutations of Wilson disease, and several clinical presentations may occur in the same family.[43] Presentation may include sardonic laughter, facial dystonia, and encephalopathy secondary to metabolic problems. Copper-colored corneal Kayser–Fleischer rings occur in about two-thirds of cases. Psychiatric features, including personality changes, affective disorders, and, infrequently, psychosis, may manifest soon after onset of Wilson disease. They can appear as the first symptom or during the course of the disease.

AUTOIMMUNE CONDITIONS

Autoimmune encephalitis comprises a group of autoimmune diseases caused by circulating autoantibodies, whose etiology is regarded as paraneoplastic or non-paraneoplastic. Psychotic symptoms often manifest early, due to anti-N-methyl-D-aspartate receptor (NMDAR) antibodies (NMDAR-Abs); in addition, later psychotic-related presentations may appear as the disease progresses. Other examples of autoimmune encephalitis are related to anti-α-amino-3-hydroxy-5-methyl-4-isoxazolepropionic acid (AMPA) receptor antibodies, anti-Caspr2 antibodies, and anti-Lgi1 antibodies. In most cases, psychiatric symptoms are the first manifestation of the disease. Some warning signs for autoimmune encephalitis in patients with progressive subacute psychiatric disease and little or no response to psychoactive drugs are reduced consciousness, disorientation, memory deficits, catatonia, autonomic dysfunction, hyponatremia, and other associated autoimmune diseases. In the presence of any of these alarm signals, evaluation should be expanded with structural imaging (magnetic resonance imaging [MRI]), serum antibodies, electroencephalogram, and lumbar puncture with cerebrospinal fluid (CSF) analysis.

Several neuropsychiatric manifestations may occur in SLE (lupus). Psychosis is more frequent in male SLE subjects and has been reported in prospective studies to vary from 0% to 17%.[44] Current evidence supports the association of psychotic symptoms with lupus-specific autoantibodies,[44] although clinic usefulness is impeded by low sensitivity.[45] Delusions or hallucinations are most common early on, but can also occur later. Typically, SLE patients will exhibit signs, symptoms, and laboratory abnormalities of systemic disease, including renal, hematologic, and pulmonary function. In addition, mood disorders, cognitive dysfunction, and encephalopathy syndrome may occur.

ALCOHOL, MEDICATION-RELATED CAUSES

Psychotic-related features can be found in acute conditions involving chronic alcohol consumption, usually following the depletion of intracellular thiamine (vitamin B1). Wernicke encephalopathy (WE) is a severe complication associated with death in 20% of patients, along with a high proportion of long-term brain damage (75%). During WE, acute brain disease caused by severe abstinence, ophthalmoplegia, gait disturbance, and mental confusion may occur. When the complications of WE are not adequately addressed, the chronic condition tends to progress to the impairment of executive functions and altered memory and language that characterize Korsakoff syndrome.[46] Additional potential causes or contributors to alcohol-related psychosis include comorbid substance abuse, alcohol-dependent withdrawal early stage, advanced age, and alcoholic idiosyncratic intoxication.

Consistent evidence has related the use of cannabis (particularly with high-concentration Tetrahydrocannabinol [THC]) to new psychotic episodes and eventual development of schizophrenia or schizophreniform disorder.[47] The causality of this association is not clear. Sympathomimetics, such as amphetamine, cause euphoria and racing thoughts, and can also produce hallucinations and delusions similar to paranoid schizophrenia. This can persist between episodes of intoxication.

High doses of steroids can produce a condition with symptoms of mood disorders, psychosis, and delirium that rapidly shift. In SLE, the so-called steroid psychosis may represent an increased risk for acute confusional state and a threefold increased risk for death.[48] In particular, steroids can also trigger an episode of mania in patients with bipolar I disorder. Use of or intoxication by other licit and illicit drugs should also be considered in the differential diagnosis of secondary psychosis.

Iatrogenic psychotic episodes may also be consequent to the continuous use or abrupt discontinuation of anticonvulsive therapy, including the first-generation ethosuximide, phenytoin, carbamazepine, valproic acid phenobarbital, and primidone as well as newer agents, such as vigabatrin, topiramate, levetiracetam, lacosamide, pregabalin, and parampanel.[27] Acute withdrawal from benzodiazepines is very often tied to acute neuropsychiatric manifestations, including psychotic symptoms.[27]

Diagnosis

DIFFERENTIAL DIAGNOSIS

The initial therapeutic approach must take into consideration the multiple factors that differentiate the clinical picture of medical illness related psychoses in distinct age groups, particularly between young adults and the elderly.

Management of primary or secondary psychosis can be complicated by multiple issues (Fig. 9.1).[49] One must carefully observe the cause-effect and temporal windows linking delusions, hallucinations, and other psychotic features with the onset timing of a medical comorbidity. Among the elderly, there is a risk of comorbidity with dementia syndromes such as FTD and Alzheimer dementia.[50] Misdiagnosis of FTD for AD may often occur, even though there is much less literature discussion.[50] In addition, a closer association of cerebrovascular risk factors and white matter hyperintensities has been reported in late-onset psychosis.[51]

The occurrence of psychoses comorbid with other clinical disease has been long described in the medical literature. Psychiatric comorbidities can affect, for instance, up to 95% of multiple sclerosis (MS) patients along the illness course and are considered a core pathology of the disease.[52] The similarity of psychiatric symptoms in MS to those observed in nonorganic psychiatric disorders makes it even more challenging for psychiatrists to differentiate between the two conditions. However, this scenario could be avoided if physicians rely on some red flags in the history and physical exam: late-onset psychiatric symptoms despite negative personal or family history of psychiatric diseases; and little or no benefit from psychiatric medications.[52] These findings should further prompt diagnostic reappraisal in patients with potential MS symptoms. In other words, the response of MS patients to psychiatric medications is poor compared to those with pure psychiatric disorders.[52,53]

In patients over 50 years old, clinical examination includes a rigorous neurologic examination, where focal signs and changes in primitive reflexes (glabellar, palmar, and snout) are observed (Table 9.5).

TABLE 9.5 ■ Laboratory Workup for Medical Psychosis

A. Hemogram and biochemical evaluation with white and red blood cells, platelets, PCR, blood glucose, electrolytes, liver and renal function, urine drug screen, thyroid testing (Free T4 and thyroid stimulating hormone (TSH)), hepatitis serologic testing, rapid plasm screening, AIDS screening, serum ferritin, transferrin saturation, toxicologic investigation.

B. Neuroimaging: cranial computed tomography, structural magnetic resonance

C. Lumbar puncture

D. Specific serology for arboviruses, encephalitis (herpes simplex, flavivirus, zika, acute disseminated encephalomyelitis, autoimmune), lupus, Lyme disease, demyelinating disorders

E. Vitamin B12, folic acid, thiamine deficiency testing

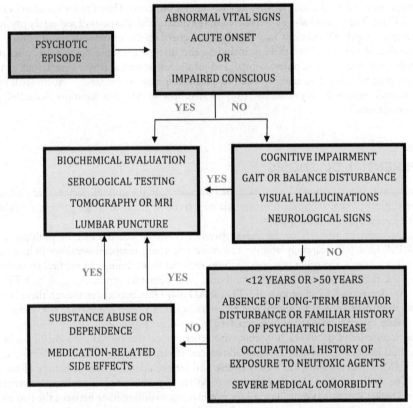

Fig. 9.2 Algorithm for psychotic episode investigation.

Exposure over years to pesticides (e.g., carbamates, Dichlorodiphenyltrichloroethane [DDT], glyphosate, organochlorines) or metals (e.g., organic lead, manganese, arsenic) may be related to the occurrence of hallucinations, aggression, and psychosis. Travel history and exposure to arbovirus epidemic areas may increase suspicion of encephalitis. In a SLE (lupus) patient who has already been diagnosed, it is important to differentiate whether the acute psychosis is due to lupus psychosis or to corticosteroid use, which can also trigger acute episodes of psychosis. Careful history will help determine the time courses of disease and corticosteroid use, and also to evaluate the need for a change in the therapeutic regimen (Figs. 9.2 and 9.3).

It is important to remember that psychoses are commonly misattributed to alcohol (and other substances), when the underlying causality is actually neurologic, medical, or psychiatric. Thoroughly reviewing the patient's history of clinical symptoms, development and course, and other relevant personal and family history information can enhance determination of true causality for alcohol-related psychosis.

The occurrence of organic psychosis in autoimmune conditions, such as anti-NMDA receptor encephalitis, may be suspected in intensively acute presentations, usually lasting from 5 to 14 days, often accompanied by viral-like features including lethargy, headache, upper respiratory symptoms, nauseas, diarrhea, and myalgia.[54] In these cases, behavioral changes are usually followed by overt neurologic symptoms, including cognitive deterioration, speech or balance disturbances, and confusional states.[54] Brain MRI with abnormal signs in Fluid-attenuated inversion recovery

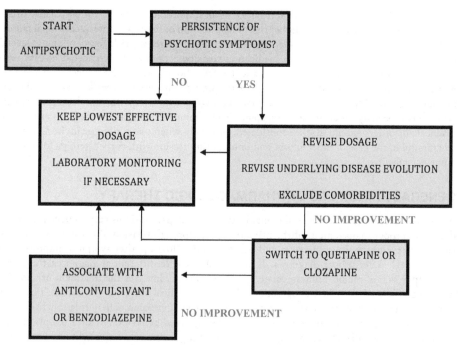

Fig. 9.3 General principles of antipsychotic treatment in illness-related psychosis.

(FLAIR) and moderate lymphocytic pleocytosis with increased protein are frequent findings, and in 60% of patients, CSF-specific oligoclonal bands are found.[55]

The clinical picture in seizure-related psychosis may closely resemble primary schizophrenic disorders, although TLE may manifest uncommon features, such as preserved affect, absence of withdrawn attitude, and visual hallucinations.[27] Among interictal psychosis (besides personality preservation, absence of negative symptoms, and a better premorbid condition), delusions and hallucination may appear less bizarre and even understandable to the clinician. In postsurgical anterior-temporal lobe resections, they occur in 3% to 10% of cases. In post-ictal psychosis, mental state includes depressed consciousness, disorientation, or delirium. Psychotic symptoms in these conditions may arise during the confusional state or present days later.[27]

Another consideration is that the first-episode psychosis among the younger elderly may often be mislabeled as depression.[56] A careful medical examination should be conducted to identify symptoms, comorbidities, and differential diagnoses. Behavioral disturbances may warrant immediate administration of pharmacologic agents, even before the comprehensive psychiatric assessment can be undertaken, to ensure the patient's safety.[57]

Some basic guidelines for interviewing acutely psychotic patients are included near the end of Chapter 1.

POTENTIAL RISKS AND COMPLICATIONS PRIOR TO THERAPY

Attention should be paid to the occurrence of a pre-morbid history of psychosis. The onset of progression to psychotic symptoms is determinant. Young adults often have psychotic symptoms after exposure to marijuana, cocaine, synthetic psychedelics, ecstasy, and other drugs. The rapid progression of symptoms can be seen in acute intoxication or cerebrovascular disease.

In older adults, age itself has been regarded as an important risk factor for psychiatric drug-associated side effects, including higher risk of falls and hip or femur fractures, acute renal failure, and Parkinson-like symptoms. Older adults are thus at increased risk for developing several adverse reactions, mostly related to medication toxicity, presence of a comorbid disease process, and use of multiple medications. Patient safety should be a major concern. Medication management requires monitoring of safe therapeutic serum levels, as well as rapidly detecting side effects.[58] Older subjects are among the higher-risk groups for developing metabolic syndrome, especially when using olanzapine or clozapine.[59] The risk for medication-induced psychotic disorders should also be considered, especially when using rifampicin, isoniazid, and ethambutol in the case of tuberculosis, and immunosuppression with corticosteroids for autoimmune encephalitis.

GENERAL PRINCIPLES OF PHARMACOLOGIC THERAPY

Successful treatment of illness- and medication-related psychosis usually depends on early diagnosis, proper management of the primary cause, thorough revision of current medications, careful interventions weighing risks and benefits, and follow-up after symptom improvement (see Fig. 9.1). After proper diagnosis, discarding all possible differential diagnoses, the therapeutic approach of medical illness–related psychoses mainly involves the treatment of underlying causes (Table 9.6). Close cooperation with other medical specialties is critical. The main targets of drug treatment are control of symptoms such as aggression, self-mutilation, hallucinations, delusions, psychomotor agitation, grossly disorganized behavior, suicide attempts, disorientation, and sleep disorders, among others contributing to increased morbidity and mortality (see Table 9.1).

Benefits and risks of morbidity and mortality should always be weighed, as several studies suggest that antipsychotic treatment is associated with increased stroke risk in the general population (Table 9.7).[60] No consensus exists on the greater efficacy of one class of antipsychotics alone compared to the others, although newer second-generation antipsychotics seem to exhibit lower vascular risks than first-generation drugs regardless of age.[61] Besides the most favorable profile of side effects, atypical antipsychotics present similar efficacy to typical agents. The use of antipsychotics should be initiated at minimal doses, and titration should be cautious in order to use the lowest dose required. The patient should be periodically reassessed regarding the need for maintenance of antipsychotic therapy, which should remain as short as possible.[62] If anticipated benefit does not occur, reevaluation of medication choice and clinical indication is recommended.

In cerebrovascular disease with psychosis, antipsychotics remain a core pharmacotherapy, as there is little evidence that other forms of medication are effective in this circumstance.[60] It is important to characterize the extent of the lesions and their nature with resonance imaging.

TABLE 9.6 ■ Therapeutic Targets of Illness- and Medication-related Psychosis

Therapeutic targets of illness- and medication-related psychosis	
• Heteroaggressiveness	• Sensoperceptive disturbances
• Self-injurious behavior	• Delusions
• Disorganized behavior	• Negative symptoms
• Sleep disorder	• Disorientation
• Suicide risk	• Psychomotor agitation

TABLE 9.7 ■ Groups Requiring Greater Caution in the Use of Antipsychotics

Clinical groups in which antipsychotic use requires greater caution	
• Advanced age with or without cognitive decline	• Suicide attempts associated with antipsychotic use
• Weakened or hospitalized patients	• Intellectual disability patients
• Presence of multiple comorbidities, particularly cardiovascular and metabolic diseases	• Evidence of malignant neuroleptic syndrome and/or serotonergic syndrome.
• Evidence of parkinsonism or dyskinetic symptoms	• Presence of auditory or visual deficit

Persistent and long-lasting psychosis may require continuous treatment, particularly in widespread cerebrovascular disease.[60] For AD, currently available treatments are symptomatic and should be started early. Clinicians should carefully evaluate the severity of behavioral symptoms, particularly when accompanied by important caregiver distress. Non-pharmacologic measures are of first choice in the management of these symptoms, and medications used to treat cognitive symptoms may also be useful in behavioral symptoms. This is the case of acetylcholinesterase inhibitors, generally indicated in all stages of the disease, while memantine (NMDA antagonist) is preferred in moderate to severe stages. Antipsychotics should be used when there is agitation associated with psychotic symptoms.[63]

Anticonvulsants may be used in patients with symptoms of mania, impulsivity, lability, or episodes of severe aggression. They should be prescribed as a second- or third-line attempt. In LBD, galantamine treatment can reduce behavioral disorders, especially visual hallucinations and nocturnal behaviors, in treated subjects compared to placebo.[64] If antipsychotic treatment is required in LBD or other Parkinson-related syndromes (i.e., severe psychosis, agitation), clozapine or quetiapine usually exhibit a more favorable profile in terms of extrapyramidal effects than other atypical drugs; in such circumstances, the lowest effective dose should be used.

Some organic psychoses may be related to diseases with rapidly progressive changes. Among them: prionic diseases, such as Creutzfeldt-Jakob disease; infectious diseases, such as herpetic encephalitis, HIV encephalitis, Lyme disease (in endemic regions), fungal infections, Whipple disease; toxic metabolic conditions, such as WE, thyroid disease, and heavy metal poisoning; autoimmune and immune-mediated diseases, such as limbic encephalitis and NMDA-abs encephalitis; genetic diseases, such as Wilson disease; and neoplastic diseases including both primary tumors and metastases. In all these cases, antipsychotic treatment is usually conducted in a hospital setting and may be administered intravenously. Cardiac monitoring is also important because of the risk of arrhythmias and other complications. Preferably, the doses should be increased gradually, according to tolerability and clinical response.

In elderly individuals, the use of potentially iatrogenic drugs, such as hypnotic medications with anticholinergic effects, should be actively reconsidered. Commonly prescribed anticholinergic medications include prednisone, prednisolone, tricyclic antidepressants, digoxin, nifedipine, antipsychotics, furosemide, ranitidine, isosorbide dinitrate, warfarin, dipyridamole, codeine, captopril, oxybutynin, and scopolamine. Simply discontinuing some of these medications may effect symptomatic improvement of the condition.

In addition, treatment with antipsychotics may have side effects, for instance weight gain, diabetes, and metabolic syndrome, in most cases requiring lab monitoring. Thus, an additional benefit of correct diagnosis of underlying medical conditions will improve prognosis for social as well as medical and psychiatric factors.

Box 9.1 Fictional Case

PART I

Mrs. Andrews, 61, presented to the emergency department with her two sons, in acute agitation. Relatives report absence of previous psychiatric history and describe the patient as "very active." During the evaluation, the patient shows great psychomotor restlessness, getting up for several moments in the chair. Asked about what would make her uneasy, she replied: "This all disgrace for envy!" According to the eldest son, the patient had never displayed depressive or psychotic symptoms. She was medicated 1 month ago by a General Practitioner [GP] with risperidone 1 mg/day, then increased to 4 mg about 2 weeks later, with some initial improvement. However, in the last week, there was substantial worsening of sleep, with more exaggerated humor and bizarre behavior (shouting out the window for neighbors "to leave her in peace and take care of their own lives"). Neurologic examination, including pupil reflex, gait, and tonus, appeared normal, but family members reported "urinary incontinence 2 days ago." Due to these symptoms, a battery of biochemistry, lumbar puncture, and neuroimaging exams were requested to rule out medical disease.

PART II

The Cerebrospinal fluid [CSF] analysis revealed pleocytosis with lymphocytic predominance and moderate elevation of protein (58 mg/dL). Widespread areas of hyperintensities were observed in the temporal, parietal, and occipital lobes in the T2 images, suggesting encephalitis of viral etiology. CSF-PCR testing confirmed the diagnosis of herpes simplex virus type 1 (HSV-1) with predominant organic psychotic presentation. Untreated HSV-1 is associated with high mortality rate (above 70%) with a reported incidence of 2 per 250,000 cases per year. When optimal treatment is implemented, mortality rates are decreased to lower than 29%. Patient was treated successfully with intravenous dosages of acyclovir for 21 days, and the antipsychotic risperidone was successfully discontinued after 15 days of hospitalization.

Summary

Medical illness related psychosis and medication-induced psychosis encompass a wide range of medical conditions associated with greater comorbidity, treatment delay, and increasing health costs. Diagnostic workup usually requires a thorough clinical and complementary investigation including careful medical exam and serologic, biochemical, and neuroimaging procedures. Medication-induced psychosis and autoimmune disease are frequently reported in distinct age groups. Early diagnosis and the correct recognition of red-flag symptoms and signs may improve the accuracy of diagnosis and guide the clinician to prompt treatment.

References

1. American Psychological Association. *The Diagnostic and Statistical Manual of Mental Disorders.* 2013; (5th ed.), Arlington, VA: Author.

2. Sciolla N. Iatrogenic psychoses. *Semin Clin Neuropsychiatry.* 1998;3:61–69.

3. Giannitelli M, Consoli A, Raffin M, et al. An overview of medical risk factors for childhood psychosis: implications for research and treatment. *Schizophr Res.* 2018;192:39–49. https://doi.org/10.1016/j.schres.2017.05.011.

4. Oskarsdottir S. Incidence and prevalence of the 22q11 deletion syndrome: a population-based study in Western Sweden. *Arch Dis Child.* 2004;89:148–151. https://doi.org/10.1136/adc.2003.026880.

5. Kales HC, Gitlin LN, Lyketsos CG. Assessment and management of behavioral and psychological symptoms of dementia. *BMJ.* 2015;350:h369.

6. Lyketsos CG, Carrillo MC, Ryan JM, et al. Neuropsychiatric symptoms in Alzheimer's disease. *Alzheimers Dement J Alzheimers Assoc.* 2011;7:532–539. https://doi.org/10.1016/j.jalz.2011.05.2410.

7. Rosenberg PB, Nowrangi MA, Lyketsos CG. Neuropsychiatric symptoms in Alzheimer's disease: what might be associated brain circuits? *Mol Aspects Med.* 2015;43–44:25–37. https://doi.org/10.1016/j.mam.2015.05.005.

8. Assal F, Cummings JL. Neuropsychiatric symptoms in the dementias. *Curr Opin Neurol.* 2002;15:445–450.

9. Pinto T, Lanctôt KL, Herrmann N. Revisiting the cholinergic hypothesis of behavioral and psychological symptoms in dementia of the Alzheimer's type. *Ageing Res Rev.* 2011;10:404–412. https://doi.org/10.1016/j.arr.2011.01.003.

10. Banno K, Nakaaki S, Sato J, et al. Neural basis of three dimensions of agitated behaviors in patients with Alzheimer disease. *Neuropsychiatr Dis Treat.* 2014;10:339–348. https://doi.org/10.2147/NDT.S57522.

11. Hirono N, Kitagaki H, Kazui H, et al. Impact of white matter changes on clinical manifestation of Alzheimer's disease: a quantitative study. *Stroke J Cereb Circ.* 2000;31:2182–2188.

12. Lee GJ, Lu PH, Hua X, et al. Depressive symptoms in mild cognitive impairment predict greater atrophy in Alzheimer's disease-related regions. *Biol Psychiatry.* 2012;71:814–821. https://doi.org/10.1016/j.biopsych.2011.12.024.

13. Mega MS, Lee L, Dinov ID, et al. Cerebral correlates of psychotic symptoms in Alzheimer's disease. *J Neurol Neurosurg Psychiatry.* 2000;69:167–171.

14. Palmqvist S, Sarwari A, Wattmo C, et al. Association between subcortical lesions and behavioral and psychological symptoms in patients with Alzheimer's disease. *Dement Geriatr Cogn Disord.* 2011;32:417–423. https://doi.org/10.1159/000335778.

15. Rafii MS, Taylor CS, Kim HT, et al. Neuropsychiatric symptoms and regional neocortical atrophy in mild cognitive impairment and Alzheimer's disease. *Am J Alzheimers Dis Other Demen.* 2014;29:159–165. https://doi.org/10.1177/1533317513507373.

16. Whitehead D, Tunnard C, Hurt C, et al. Frontotemporal atrophy associated with paranoid delusions in women with Alzheimer's disease. *Int Psychogeriatr IPA.* 2012;24:99–107. https://doi.org/10.1017/S1041610211000974.

17. Poulin SP, Dautoff R, Morris JC, et al. Amygdala atrophy is prominent in early Alzheimer's disease and relates to symptom severity. *Psychiatry Res.* 2011;194:7–13. https://doi.org/10.1016/j.pscychresns.2011.06.014.

18. Trzepacz PT, Yu P, Bhamidipati PK, et al. Frontolimbic atrophy is associated with agitation and aggression in mild cognitive impairment and Alzheimer's disease. *Alzheimers Dement J Alzheimers Assoc.* 2013;9:S95–S104.e1. https://doi.org/10.1016/j.jalz.2012.10.005.

19. Tsai CF, Hung CW, Lirng JF, et al. Differences in brain metabolism associated with agitation and depression in Alzheimer's disease. *East Asian Arch Psychiatry Off J Hong Kong Coll Psychiatr Dong Ya Jing Shen Ke Xue Zhi Xianggang Jing Shen Ke Yi Xue Yuan Qi Kan.* 2013;23:86–90.

20. Rolland Y, Payoux P, Lauwers-Cances V, et al. A SPECT study of wandering behavior in Alzheimer's disease. *Int J Geriatr Psychiatry.* 2005;20:816–820. https://doi.org/10.1002/gps.1362.

21. Balthazar MLF, Pereira FRS, Lopes TM, et al. Neuropsychiatric symptoms in Alzheimer's disease are related to functional connectivity alterations in the salience network. *Hum Brain Mapp.* 2014;35:1237–1246. https://doi.org/10.1002/hbm.22248.

22. Serra L, Perri R, Cercignani M, et al. Are the behavioral symptoms of Alzheimer's disease directly associated with neurodegeneration? *J Alzheimers Dis.* 2010;21:627–639. https://doi.org/10.3233/JAD-2010-100048.

23. Donovan NJ, Wadsworth LP, Lorius N, et al. Regional cortical thinning predicts worsening apathy and hallucinations across the Alzheimer disease spectrum. *Am J Geriatr Psychiatry Off J Am Assoc Geriatr Psychiatry.* 2014;22:1168–1179. https://doi.org/10.1016/j.jagp.2013.03.006.

24. Rajkowska G, Miguel-Hidalgo JJ, Dubey P, et al. Prominent reduction in pyramidal neurons density in the orbitofrontal cortex of elderly depressed patients. *Biol Psychiatry.* 2005;58:297–306. https://doi.org/10.1016/j.biopsych.2005.04.013.

25. Eslinger PJ, Damasio AR. Severe disturbance of higher cognition after bilateral frontal lobe ablation: patient EVR. *Neurology.* 1985;35:1731–1741.

26. Bear DM, Fedio P. Quantitative analysis of interictal behavior in temporal lobe epilepsy. *Arch Neurol.* 1977;34:454–467. https://doi.org/10.1001/archneur.1977.00500200014003.

27. Kanner AM, Rivas-Grajales AM. Psychosis of epilepsy: a multifaceted neuropsychiatric disorder. *CNS Spectr.* 2016;21:247–257. https://doi.org/10.1017/S1092852916000250.

28. Gallhofer B, Trimble MR, Frackowiak R, et al. A study of cerebral blood flow and metabolism in epileptic psychosis using positron emission tomography and oxygen. *J Neurol Neurosurg Psychiatry.* 1985;48:201–206. https://doi.org/10.1136/jnnp.48.3.201.

29. Tighe SK, Oishi K, Mori S, et al. Diffusion tensor imaging of neuropsychiatric symptoms in mild cognitive impairment and Alzheimer's dementia. *J Neuropsychiatry Clin Neurosci.* 2012;24:484–488. https://doi.org/10.1176/appi.neuropsych.11120375.

30. Smith MJ, Thirthalli J, Abdallah AB, et al. Prevalence of psychotic symptoms in substance users: a comparison across substances. *Compr Psychiatry.* 2009;50:245–250. https://doi.org/10.1016/j.comppsych.2008.07.009.

31. Keshavan MS, Kaneko Y. Secondary psychoses: an update. *World Psychiatry.* 2013;12:4–15. https://doi.org/10.1002/wps.20001.

32. Appenzeller S, Cendes F, Costallat LTL. Acute psychosis in systemic lupus erythematosus. *Rheumatol Int.* 2008;28:237–243. https://doi.org/10.1007/s00296-007-0410-x.

33. Alves GS, Carvalho AF, de Amorim de Carvalho L, et al. Neuroimaging findings related to behavioral disturbances in Alzheimer's disease: a systematic review. *Curr Alzheimer Res.* 2017;14:61–75.

34. Eska K, Graessel E, Donath C, et al. Predictors of institutionalization of dementia patients in mild and moderate stages: a 4-year prospective analysis. *Dement Geriatr Cogn Disord Extra.* 2013;3:426–445. https://doi.org/10.1159/000355079.

35. Galvin JE. Cognitive change in Parkinson disease. *Alzheimer Dis Assoc Disord.* 2006;20:302–310. https://doi.org/10.1097/01.wad.0000213858.27731.f8.

36. Tarawneh R, Galvin J. Dementia with Lewy bodies and other synucleinopathies. In: Weiner, MF., Lipton, AM. *Textbook of Alzheimer Disease and Other Dementias.* Washington, DC: American Psychiatric Publishing; 2009; pages 195–218.

37. Ballard C, Neill D, O'Brien J, et al. Anxiety, depression and psychosis in vascular dementia: prevalence and associations. *J Affect Disord.* 2000;59:97–106. https://doi.org/10.1016/S0165-0327; (99)00057-9.

38. Corrêa-Oliveira GE, do Amaral JL, da Fonseca BAL, et al. Zika virus infection followed by a first episode of psychosis: another flavivirus leading to pure psychiatric symptomatology. *Rev Bras Psiquiatr.* 2017;39:381–382. https://doi.org/10.1590/1516-4446-2017-2308.

39. Cao-Lormeau V-M, Blake A, Mons S, et al. Guillain-Barré Syndrome outbreak associated with Zika virus infection in French Polynesia: a case-control study. *Lancet.* 2016;387:1531–1539. https://doi.org/10.1016/S0140-6736; (16)00562-6.

40. Verma A, Kumar A. Neurocysticercosis presenting as acute psychosis: a rare case report from rural India. *Asian J Psychiatry.* 2013;6:611–613. https://doi.org/10.1016/j.ajp.2013.06.008.

41. Urias-Uribe L, Valdez-Solis E, González-Milán C, et al. Psychosis crisis associated with thyrotoxicosis due to Graves' disease. *Case Rep Psychiatry.* 2017;2017:1–4. https://doi.org/10.1155/2017/6803682.

42. Huster D, Hoppert M, Lutsenko S, et al. Defective cellular localization of mutant ATP7B in Wilson's disease patients and hepatoma cell lines. *Gastroenterology.* 2003;124:335–345. https://doi.org/10.1053/gast.2003.50066.

43. Usta J, Wehbeh A, Rida K, et al. Phenotype-genotype correlation in Wilson disease in a large Lebanese family: association of c.2299insC with hepatic and of p. Ala1003Thr with neurologic phenotype. *PLoS One.* 2014;9:e109727. https://doi.org/10.1371/journal.pone.0109727.

44. Hanly JG, Li Q, Su L, et al. Psychosis in systemic lupus erythematosus: results from an International Inception Cohort Study. *Arthritis Rheumatol.* 2019;71:281–289. https://doi.org/10.1002/art.40764.

45. Yoshio T, Okamoto H. Diagnosis and differential diagnosis. In: Hirohata S, ed. *Neuropsychiatric Systemic Lupus Erythematosus.* Cham: Springer International Publishing; 2018:93–112. https://doi.org/10.1007/978-3-319-76496-2_7.

46. Thomson AD, Marshall EJ. The natural history and pathophysiology of Wernicke's Encephalopathy and Korsakoff's Psychosis. *Alcohol Alcohol.* 2006;41:151–158. https://doi.org/10.1093/alcalc/agh249.

47. Di Forti M, Quattrone D, Freeman TP, et al. The contribution of cannabis use to variation in the incidence of psychotic disorder across Europe (EU-GEI): a multicentre case-control study. *Lancet Psychiatry.* 2019;6:427–436. https://doi.org/10.1016/S2215-0366; (19)30048-3.

48. Abe G, Kikuchi H, Arinuma Y, et al. Brain MRI in patients with acute confusional state of diffuse psychiatric/neuropsychological syndromes in systemic lupus erythematosus. *Mod Rheumatol.* 2017;27:278–283. https://doi.org/10.1080/14397595.2016.1193966.

49. Abou-Saleh MT, Katona CLE, Kumar A. *Principles and Practice of Geriatric Psychiatry.* Chichester: John Wiley; 2011.

50. Neary D, Snowden JS, Gustafson L, et al. Frontotemporal lobar degeneration: a consensus on clinical diagnostic criteria. *Neurology.* 1998;51:1546–1554.

51. Aylward EH, Roberts-Twillie JV, Barta PE, et al. Basal ganglia volumes and white matter hyperintensities in patients with bipolar disorder. *Am J Psychiatry.* 1994;151:687–693.

52. Chalah MA, Ayache SS. Psychiatric event in multiple sclerosis: could it be the tip of the iceberg? *Rev Bras Psiquiatr.* 2017;39:365–368. https://doi.org/10.1590/1516-4446-2016-2105.
53. Hickie I, Scott E, Wilhelm K, et al. Subcortical hyperintensities on magnetic resonance imaging in patients with severe depression—a longitudinal evaluation. *Biol Psychiatry.* 1997;42:367–374. https://doi.org/10.1016/S0006-3223; (96)00363-0.
54. Kayser MS, Dalmau J. Anti-NMDA receptor encephalitis in psychiatry. *Curr Psychiatry Rev.* 2011;7:189–193. https://doi.org/10.2174/157340011797183184.
55. Dalmau J, Lancaster E, Martinez-Hernandez E, et al. Clinical experience and laboratory investigations in patients with anti-NMDAR encephalitis. *Lancet Neurol.* 2011;10:63–74. https://doi.org/10.1016/S1474-4422; (10)70253-2.
56. Sajatovic M, Herrmann N, Shulman K. Acute mania and bipolar affective disorder. In: Abou-Saleh, MT, Katona, CLE, Kumar, *Principles and Practice of Geriatric Psychiatry.* third edition, Wiley-Blackwell, pages 576–587, 2011.
57. Malhi GS, Adams D, Lampe L, et al. Clinical practice recommendations for bipolar disorder. *Acta Psychiatr Scand Suppl.* 2009;119(s439):27–46. https://doi.org/10.1111/j.1600-0447.2009.01383.x.
58. Sherrod T, Quinlan-Colwell A, Lattimore TB, et al. Older adults with bipolar disorder: guidelines for primary care providers. *J Gerontol Nurs.* 2010;36:20–27. quiz 28–29. https://doi.org/10.3928/00989134-20100108-05.
59. McIntyre RS, Danilewitz M, Liauw SS, et al. Bipolar disorder and metabolic syndrome: an international perspective. *J Affect Disord.* 2010;126:366–387. https://doi.org/10.1016/j.jad.2010.04.012.
60. Joyce EM. Organic psychosis: the pathobiology and treatment of delusions. *CNS Neurosci Ther.* 2018;24(7):598–603. https://doi.org/10.1111/cns.12973. Epub 2018 May 15. Review 29766653.
61. Hsu WT, Esmaily-Fard A, Lai CC, et al. Antipsychotics and the risk of cerebrovascular accident: a systematic review and meta-analysis of observational studies. *J Am Med Dir Assoc.* 2017;18(8):692–699. https://doi.org/10.1016/j.jamda.2017.02.020. Epub 2017 Apr 18. Review 28431909.
62. Forlenza OV, Cretaz E, Diniz BS. [The use of antipsychotics in patients with dementia]. *Braz J Psychiatry.* 2008;30(3):265–270. Review. Portuguese. PMID: 18833428.
63. Rockwood K, Mitnitski A, Richard M, et al. Neuropsychiatric symptom clusters targeted for treatment at earlier versus later stages of dementia. *Int J Geriatr Psychiatry.* 2015;30(4):357–367. https://doi.org/10.1002/gps.4136. Epub 2014 May 5. 24798635.
64. Cummings JL, Schneider L, Tariot PN, et al. Reduction of behavioral disturbances and caregiver distress by galantamine in patients with Alzheimer's disease. *Am J Psychiatry.* 2004;161(3):532–538.

Note: Page numbers followed by *f* indicate figures, *t* indicate tables and *b* indicate boxes.